Pluralism in Counselling and Psychotherapy

This book explores the concept of pluralism in therapy, emphasising the value of multiple therapeutic approaches. It introduces 'pluralistic therapy', developed by Mick Cooper and John McLeod, as a response to divisions in the therapy field, particularly the dominance of CBT and medicalised models.

Within its chapters, the philosophical roots of pluralism are discussed, which, when applied to therapy, encourage drawing from multiple approaches in contrast to a monistic attitude, which promotes using singular approaches 'purely': the therapeutic relationship is emphasised as more important to outcomes than specific approaches or techniques. The political meanings of pluralism are also examined, especially in relation to regulation, professional identity, and the impact of political and professional power structures on therapists' practices. The book also critiques increasingly standardised 'treatments', AI therapy, and rigid research methodologies, advocating for a more inclusive, relational, and flexible attitude towards the practice and provision of therapy.

Addressing contemporary challenges such as the SCoPEd framework, the rise of AI, and the resurgence of psychedelic therapies, the book ultimately argues that a philosophically and politically informed pluralism is essential for a brighter future for the therapy professions and their diversity of therapies, therapists, and clients. This is an essential read for any therapist or mental health practitioner who is interested in learning more about pluralistic approaches to therapy.

Jay Beichman is a writer, counsellor and psychotherapist living and working in Brighton in the UK. He has been qualified and in practice in a variety of contexts since 1998.

'An invigorating, informed, critical exploration of the role and meaning of pluralism in therapy. Jay Beichman goes beyond the pluralistic approach developed by John McLeod and myself, to look at the wider implications of pluralistic thinking and practice for the field of counselling and psychotherapy. A valuable contribution that can sharpen our work.'

Mick Cooper, *Professor of Counselling Psychology,*
University of Roehampton

'The philosophical lens of pluralism in counselling and psychotherapy has gained much traction over the last few years, informing thinking and shaping practice. In this wonderful text, Beichman undertakes a detailed and compelling account of its scope across therapy, philosophy, practice and broader social justice considerations. For anyone interested in a critical discussion of the key philosophical developments that underpin our work – and who wouldn't be – this book brings much to the table and is highly recommended, for practitioners, academics, theorists and broader social scientists alike.'

Andrew Reeves, *Professor in Counselling Professions and*
Mental Health, University of Chester, UK, and Senior Accredited
Counsellor/Psychotherapist and Coach

'This book is a great contribution to the fields of counselling, psychotherapy, philosophy, politics and policy. It provides a wide exploration of pluralism and its implications for therapeutic practice and policy. It explores the historical, philosophical, and political dimensions of pluralistic therapy, and provides a convincing analysis of how diverse approaches can coexist and complement one another. The book critically examines key debates, including professionalisation, regulation, and the dominance of the medical model, making it a unique resource for practitioners, researchers, and students alike. Insightful and rigorously argued, written in an accessible language, this beautiful book challenges rigid frameworks and advocates for a more flexible, socially just, and inclusive approach to therapy.'

Sophia Balamoutsou, PhD, *Coach, Counsellor, Researcher, Trainer,*
Institute of Agri-Food and Life Sciences (Agro-Health) Hellenic
Mediterranean University Research Centre, Heraklion, Crete, Greece

'It is great to see a new voice critiquing how pluralistic approaches might inform the therapy professions. Jay Beichman brings an insightful critique that will be invaluable to trainees, trainers, supervisors and experienced practitioners seeking to explore and better understand pluralistic lenses (conceptual and practice-based). Importantly, Jay brings a maverick edge to considerations – and it's essential that we have such innovative and challenging voices supporting advancement of the therapy professions.'

Lynne Gabriel, OBE, *Professor of Counselling and Mental Health*
at York St John University, UK, and BACP President

Pluralism in Counselling and Psychotherapy

Philosophy, Politics, and Practice

Jay Beichman

Routledge
Taylor & Francis Group

LONDON AND NEW YORK

Designed cover image: Hexagon motion concept – stock illustration.
MUDESIGN/DigitalVision Vectors via Getty Images.

First published 2026
by Routledge
4 Park Square, Milton Park, Abingdon, Oxon OX14 4RN

and by Routledge
605 Third Avenue, New York, NY 10158

*Routledge is an imprint of the Taylor & Francis Group, an informa
business*

© 2026 Jay Beichman

British Library Cataloguing-in-Publication Data
A catalogue record for this book is available from the British Library

ISBN: 978-1-032-74241-0 (hbk)
ISBN: 978-1-032-72317-4 (pbk)
ISBN: 978-1-003-46833-2 (ebk)

DOI: 10.4324/9781003468332

Typeset in Times New Roman
by KnowledgeWorks Global Ltd.

Contents

Foreword

In the ever-evolving landscape of counselling and psychotherapy, the concept of pluralism emerges as a beacon of inclusivity and adaptability. Jay Beichman's *Pluralism in Counselling and Psychotherapy: Philosophy, Politics, and Practice* offers an exploration of this concept, advocating for a therapeutic field that values multiple approaches and resists the dominance of any single methodology.

As those who, like me, identify with pluralism strive to 'lean in' and evolve their thinking, this book deepens the ways that we can think about our theoretical and ethical positioning when we are at risk of simply creating another model of therapy. Beichman argues that the use of pluralism as a way of thinking about therapy is of value to all practitioners within our discipline, and he looks at how the contemporary and historical approaches to therapy have led us to the current state of play and the tensions this has produced between the 'art' and 'science' of therapeutic endeavours. Using a pluralistic approach to bridge the politics and context of therapeutic practice, the variety of therapeutic practices which are undertaken, and the professionals themselves, he broadens the frame of thinking and actively addresses some of the key challenges we face.

By drawing away from the 'how to?' to the 'why?', Beichman resurfaces the defining elements of pluralistic thinking. He argues that the world of counselling and psychotherapy is pluralistic by nature and that this is a strength – not a weakness – and an inherent dimension of the therapy world. This plurality is found in the variety of practitioners and the approaches they take to respond to client problems in living, the variety of ways clients experience their lives, and their need to accommodate contemporary working contexts.

This book is written in such a way that the author accompanies us through some of the key information we need to understand contemporary therapy and the challenges we face – starting with an exploration of the origins of pluralistic philosophy and how the application of pluralism to political systems serves to enhance social justice and power imbalance. Beichman also points to the ubiquity and uniformity of cognitive behavioural approaches in modern mental healthcare to argue that we can instead strive to flexibly collaborate according to individual client needs and engage with one another to combine the 'being with' and the 'doing with' aspects of practice.

The beginning chapter sets the stage by defining pluralism and its application to therapy, particularly within the contexts of the UK and the USA. It highlights the importance of embracing diverse therapeutic approaches, situating Mick Cooper and John McLeod's pluralistic therapy as a potentially pivotal response to the divisions within the field. Chapter 2 delves into the historical development of therapy, tracing its evolution from Freud's psychoanalysis to contemporary pluralistic approaches. It underscores the impact of research methodologies, particularly randomised controlled trials, on the field's development and highlights the ongoing debates over the distinctions between counselling and psychotherapy. Cooper and McLeod's pluralistic therapy is examined in detail in the context of therapy history.

Chapter 3 explores the philosophical underpinnings of pluralism, tracing its roots from ancient Greek thinkers to modern philosophers like William James and Emmanuel Levinas. This chapter challenges the dominance of rigid single approaches in therapy, advocating for a more flexible and collaborative attitude. It also distinguishes between cultural pluralism and multiculturalism, relating these concepts to the therapy field's preference for dominant models.

Chapter 4 examines the intersection of pluralism and politics, exploring how power dynamics influence therapy's professionalisation and regulation. It critiques the assumption that democracy is genuinely pluralistic and applies Connolly's ideas about micropolitics and macropolitics to the therapy field. This chapter also challenges research politics and entrenched research methodologies, advocating for the recognition of qualitative and practitioner-based evidence.

The fifth chapter explores the relationship between therapeutic approaches and practitioner identities, a further layer of plurality and politics, while also considering the growing influence of artificial intelligence. Given this landscape, Chapter 6 delves into the importance of, and evidence for, flexibility in therapy. It emphasises client collaboration and adaptable methods over rigid, single-approach models. A turn to an ethic-driven rather than model-driven approach leads Beichman to propose that we think about therapy within a flexibility–rigidity continuum, highlighting the limitations imposed by public health systems that favour standardised interventions. Chapter 7 then reminds us that 'It's the Relationship, Stupid', and underscores the central role of the therapeutic relationship in psychotherapy. It argues that relational factors are more critical to therapy's success than specific techniques, highlighting that despite this strong evidence supporting the importance of the therapeutic relationship, the field remains dominated by evidence-based, technique-driven models like CBT. This chapter advocates for creative collaboration between therapists and clients, emphasising the necessity of human connection.

Chapter 8, 'Therapy Wars', reflects on how we got to this place of dissensus within the profession and examines the historical and ongoing conflicts within the therapy field. It explores the divide between scientific/medical approaches and more intuitive, relational models. The chapter argues that pluralistic therapy emerged as a response to these divisions, recognising the validity of multiple therapeutic approaches. It suggests that these conflicts, while reflective of competitiveness and ideological differences, can contribute positively to the profession's evolution and capacity to respond to a range of client needs and presentations. Chapter 9 responds to this by exploring metacommunication, or 'talking about talking', as a core practice in therapy, which allows us to incorporate the range of ways of working in the light of our underlying priority to fit therapy to the client and not the model. It emphasises collaboration and shared decision-making between therapists and clients, which allows therapy to be tailored to individual needs. The chapter discusses the historical and theoretical foundations of metacommunication, its role in addressing power dynamics, and its potential to resolve professional disputes within therapy. It argues that metacommunication can strengthen the therapeutic relationship and challenge rigid, medicalised approaches to therapy.

Because we are being guided through a pluralistic approach to therapy, we are being invited to live with uncertainty about what we do, and in Chapter 10, 'Uncertainty, Understanding, Modernism, and Postmodernism', Beichman explores the tension between uncertainty and understanding in therapy. It highlights how therapists and clients navigate ambiguity, balancing the need for structured models with the acceptance of unpredictability. The chapter critiques the pressure for certainty in therapy research and healthcare systems, arguing that rigidity can constrain creative and personalised therapeutic encounters. It suggests embracing uncertainty can lead to a more adaptable and effective therapeutic practice. To reinforce this position, Chapter 11, about the common factors approach in psychotherapy, traces its origins from Rosenzweig's 1936 paper to contemporary models, suggesting effective therapy stems from shared elements across modalities, such as the therapeutic relationship, client expectations, and structured intervention, rather than approach-specific techniques. The chapter explores different integrative approaches – common factors, theoretical integration, and technical eclecticism – contrasting them with pluralism, which values therapeutic diversity without wishing for unification. A dialectical pluralism is proposed, balancing integration with recognising irreducible differences to ensure psychotherapy remains adaptable and inclusive.

The book concludes by exploring the evolving landscape of therapy, focusing on professionalisation, regulation, and the impact of pluralism on the field's future. The push for statutory regulation is critiqued as to whether it genuinely protects clients or simply reinforces hierarchical structures. The controversial SCoPEd framework is examined as a regulatory tool that risks favouring medicalised approaches while marginalising relational therapies. The book advocates for a therapeutic landscape that values diversity and collaboration over rigid frameworks, emphasising that the future of therapy depends on resisting homogenisation and embracing pluralism.

Throughout the book, Beichman explores the tensions that exist for therapists, many of which emerge from an apparent inability to navigate the plurality of our profession. Beichman's work is a clarion call for the therapy field to embrace pluralism in its philosophical, political, and practical dimensions. By valuing diverse therapeutic approaches and resisting homogenisation, we can create a more inclusive and adaptable therapeutic landscape that honours both client autonomy and the richness of therapeutic diversity. This book is an essential read for anyone committed to advancing the field of counselling and psychotherapy in a way that truly reflects the complexity and diversity of human experience.

Professor Kate Smith, Co-editor of *Pluralistic Practice*,
Head of Department of Mental Health and Wellbeing,
School of Education, University of Aberdeen

Abbreviations

ACP	Alliance for Counselling and Psychotherapy
ACT	Acceptance and Commitment Therapy
AHP	Association of Humanistic Psychology
AI	Artificial Intelligence
AIT	AI Therapy
APA	American Psychological Association
BACP	British Association for Counselling and Psychotherapy
BMRC	British Medical Research Council
BPC	British Psychoanalytic Council
BPS	British Psychological Society
CBT	Cognitive Behavioural Therapy
CORE	Clinical Outcomes in Routine Evaluation
COSCA	Counselling and Psychotherapy in Scotland
CPCAB	Counselling and Psychotherapy Central Awarding Body
CPD	Continuing professional development
DH	Department of Health
DSM	Diagnostic and Statistical Manual of Mental Disorders
EAP	Employee Assistance Programme
EBP	Evidence-based practice
EMDR	Eye Movement Desensitisation and Reprocessing
EST	Empirically supported treatment
GAD	Generalised Anxiety Disorder
HPC	Health Professions Council
IAPT	Increasing Access to Psychological Therapies
JPI	Journal of Psychotherapy Integration
MBCT	Mindfulness-Based Cognitive Therapy
MTC	Meta-therapeutic communication
NCPS	The National Counselling and Psychotherapy Society
NHS	National Health Service
NHSTT	National Health Service Talking Therapies
NICE	National Institute for Health and Care Excellence (previously National Institute for Clinical Excellence)

NPM	New Public Management
PBE	Practice-based evidence
PCA	Person-Centred Approach
PCSR	Psychotherapists and Counsellors for Social Responsibility
PCU	Psychotherapy and Counselling Union
PLG	Professional Liaison Group
PSA	Professional Standards Authority for Health and Social Care
PTSD	post-traumatic stress disorder
PWP	Psychological Wellbeing Practitioner
RCP	Royal College of Psychiatrists
RCT	randomised controlled trial
REBT	Rational Emotional Behaviour Therapy
SCoPEd	Scope of Practice and Education
SEMI	Severe and Enduring Mental Illnesses
SEPI	Society for the Exploration of Psychotherapy Integration
SPR	Society for Psychotherapy Research
SR	statutory regulation
TA	Transactional Analysis
TT	Talking Therapies
UKCP	United Kingdom Council for Psychotherapy

Chapter 1

Introduction

Counselling, Psychotherapy, Therapy, Clients, and Patients

One problem inherent in debates about therapy is the use of the different terms 'counselling', 'psychotherapy', and 'therapy'. For linguistic ease, and throughout this book, I will be mainly using the word 'therapy' to refer to 'counselling' and 'psychotherapy', the word 'therapist' to refer to 'counsellor' and 'psychotherapist', and the word 'therapeutic' to refer to 'psychotherapeutic'. Sometimes, for reasons of either syntax or meaning, those rules are broken. This decision is not uncontroversial: some 'counsellors' and some 'psychotherapists' insist that there are real differences in their practices, and I am not wholly unsympathetic to their arguments. However, it is arguable whether there are any essential differences between 'counselling' and 'psychotherapy': Dunnet et al. (2007) assert that there is a 'lack of any reliable evidence indicating a difference between the practices of "counselling" and "psychotherapy"'(quoted in Cooper, 2008, p. 9). This is an issue that I shall return to in later parts of this book. There is also debate and confusion about whether people who attend therapy should be called 'clients' or 'patients'. Again, I call all these people 'clients' for linguistic ease. I also own that I am doing this because of the association of the word 'patient' with the medical model, which reflects a dominant ideology that needs to be challenged in books such as this by careful use of language.

Psychological or 'talking therapy' is conceptualised and defined differently across the globe, which means that therapy is de facto a pluralistic field. There are similarities and differences between how particular nations conceptualise and, therefore, practise what they mean by 'counselling', 'psychotherapy' and 'therapy'. In the USA, because licensing varies from state to state, the pluralism of therapy conceptualisation/practice cannot be said to have a unified meaning even within its borders. This plurality of conceptualisation/practice is true even within the relatively narrow confines of the Anglosphere before one gets to the rest of the world. For instance, if we take the USA as just one example, 'counseling' (spelt with one l as opposed to two ls in the UK) is associated with school counselling, marriage counselling, rehabilitation counselling, mental health counselling, addiction counselling and career counselling (e.g. Leahy et al., 2015). Although in the early years

DOI: 10.4324/9781003468332-1

of 'counselling' in the UK it was associated with employee counselling and marriage counselling, it has now come to mean an activity much like 'psychotherapy': it is certainly not associated with giving careers advice to pupils in secondary education (even by 'school counsellors', who, in the UK, offer emotional support about psychological issues which may or may not be rooted in educational difficulties). In the USA, '[p]ractitioners typically identify first with their specialty area of practice [e.g. education or rehabilitation], and secondarily with the profession of counseling' (Leahy et al., p. 5). In the UK, the opposite is the case. Practitioners identify firstly as 'counsellors', 'psychotherapists', or 'therapists' and then qualify that, usually, with an approach such as psychodynamic, person-centred, integrative, or pluralistic. Although 'school counsellors' do like the identity of 'school counsellor' as indicative of a speciality, most therapists identify with approach over other descriptors.

Therefore, when considering therapy on an international scale, we must recognise that there is a plurality of professional and regulatory systems with direct and incontrovertible impacts on what people designate therapy to mean and how it should or should not be practised. Definitions of therapy are constantly and diversely evolving in different ways in different countries. The practices are similar but not the same. Therapy practice is always and everywhere contextually dependent and socially constructed. In the UK, the latest 'SCoPEd' crisis (about which, more later, in Chapter 12) was perhaps brought about by membership bodies trying to force through definitions of apparently different professional levels of therapeutic practice, purportedly for the benefit of members and the public. However, many members (almost 50% of one membership body allowed to vote on the matter) disagree with the definitions proposed by the alliance of these powerful membership bodies. A successful social construction needs a shared consensus, which is notoriously difficult to find in the world of therapy.

Pluralism and Pluralistic Therapy

Throughout my career, I have been particularly interested in issues raised by debates about commonalities and differences between therapeutic approaches. The publication of Cooper and McLeod's (2011) book *Pluralistic Counselling and Psychotherapy* intensified the controversy of these debates around various issues, such as whether some approaches are superior to others and whether practitioners should identify with only one approach or integrate different ones. While integrative therapy, before it, has a long history, the publication of Cooper and McLeod's book provided a focal point for a new 'pluralistic' agenda. While it may not be that established as a 'brand' outside the profession, pluralistic therapy is well known within it and has had a significant impact on professionals and their practices.

As practitioners most commonly perceive it, pluralistic therapy is a form of therapy for practice and research, first articulated by Mick Cooper and John McLeod (2007). It is a relatively recent phenomenon within the therapy world that offers some hope of bringing peace to 'wars' over different approaches (Saltzman &

Norcross, 1990). It also offers a pragmatic, research-friendly framework that might impact the provision of therapy in an era of 'evidence-based' practice, professionalisation, regulation and 'audit cultures' (e.g. King & Moutsou, 2010). Therapy is at a 'critical juncture' (Aldridge, 2011), in which counsellors and psychotherapists are often side-lined in favour of the creation of new types of paraprofessionals (e.g. Department of Health, 2008).

Therefore, the practices of counsellors and psychotherapists might become severely marginalised and devalued unless a pluralistic agenda makes some progress in the coming years. Clients also might want to access different types of therapies and/or therapists who are able and willing to work flexibly. Increasingly, different therapies and therapists, unable to gain admittance to or dismissed by the public sector, are retreating to or finding refuge in the private sector. If providers want different kinds of therapies to reach beyond the financially solvent, then the pluralistic agenda needs to gain traction. If, as it is presently articulated and presented, it is failing in this, then understandings need to be reached as to how it might be re-articulated and re-presented. Those in favour of pluralistic perspectives and/or practices need to re-articulate their ideas to convince practitioners themselves and, by proxy, providers and clients, in order to facilitate and enable the long-term survival of counselling and psychotherapy characterised by a healthy proliferation of different approaches.

'Pluralism', as a philosophy which underpins pluralistic therapy, is explored in Chapter 3. It has various meanings depending on disciplinary context; for instance, it is closely associated with multiculturalism. Although multiculturalism – one type of pluralism – does relate to developments in therapy and will be referred to in later chapters, in this book, a pluralistic approach to therapy primarily refers to tolerance towards and the promotion and practice of different therapeutic approaches. I am concerned with the impact of pluralistic approaches on therapy: for its practitioners, other stakeholders, and therapy as a practice. In this book, I often refer to pluralistic 'approaches', 'perspectives', and 'practices' because I see pluralism as something that is not 'owned' by Cooper and McLeod; simultaneously, I do recognise that when practitioners refer to 'pluralistic therapy' they are usually referring to Cooper and McLeod's approach. However, the relationship between pluralistic therapy as a practice and pluralism as a philosophy/perspective is of central importance and, to a certain extent, they are inextricably linked. So, two important questions in relation to pluralism and pluralistic therapy are: 1) What does pluralism mean? and 2) Is Mick Cooper and John McLeod's articulation of a pluralistic therapy actually pluralistic?

There are a multitude of issues that cause divisions in the psychological therapies. For instance, regulation and professionalisation, most particularly statutory regulation (SR), caused much turbulence amongst practitioners, especially when the government proposed it via the Health Professions Council (HPC) in 2004 (Aldridge, 2011). With a change of government, those proposals were shelved, and a voluntary registration scheme was introduced in its stead, but this attempt to statutorily regulate counselling and psychotherapy was controversial and divisive, and the issue of SR remains active (e.g. Department of Health, 2017; UK Parliament, 2019). Some practitioners shake their heads in dismay that the professions have not yet been statutorily regulated, while others warn that SR might be the death of therapy as we have known it. Concerns about regulation and professionalisation are explored at various points throughout this book.

The need to prove the superiority of one therapeutic approach over another has never resonated with me. From the beginning of my training in 1996, I have been aware of the 'different words for the same thing' so prevalent in therapy theories. In my first year of training, I was fortunate enough to attend a lively seminar with Petruska Clarkson. I was impressed by her framework, which articulated how therapy can be viewed as operating within five different types of relationship (Clarkson, 2003/1995). This seemed to be a coherent way of understanding therapy and how to practise it, and it made more sense than attempting to stay within one approach. Many of my colleagues identified with the person-centred emphasis of our training. However, it was a humanistic rather than a person-centred course, and I was also introduced to Gestalt therapy, Transactional Analysis (TA), existential philosophy, and other approaches; I experienced the course as an integrative one or, as I might now conceptualise it, a pluralistic one. I also saw the person of the therapist as centrally important. My path to training came from attending therapy with a private practitioner and, some way into that, having a sense that I could be a practitioner myself, a path she encouraged me to follow. I never even asked nor cared what approach she was using. At that time, what I needed and received was an empathetic practitioner who I felt genuinely cared about my life story and current confusions. She had essential generic qualities such as warmth and the ability to connect. Since I first went to that therapist in the early 1990s, valuing these simple relational qualities has been drowned out by the clamour for other ways of identifying effectiveness and efficiency. Rather than the best person for the job, providers are looking for the best 'abstract approach'.

My experience – as a client, a trainee therapist, and a qualified therapist – has led me to evaluate the quality of therapy and therapists in ways that do not align with current assumptions of how therapeutic effectiveness should be researched. A common critique of pluralism, as with integrative therapy before it, is that it proposes that 'all should have prizes' and signifies, perhaps, a defensive posture that cannot tolerate ideas of 'winners and losers' or 'better and worse'. I accept that there may be better and worse therapy; I do not accept that 'better' and 'worse' can be located within approaches. I believe there are better and worse therapists, so clients are best advised to look for who rather than what.

So, I accept the spirit, if not the letter, of the pluralistic approach. I value its strengths while being aware of its weaknesses. I accept that it offers some solutions, but many problems regarding therapy theories, practices and research remain unresolved.

I have always been fascinated by what influences therapists to become therapists. Although this is seemingly unconnected to the phenomena of pluralism and therapy, this book is also about the deeply felt and embodied experience of being a therapist and how therapists practise in the light of all their personal and professional experiences. The argument for a more pluralistic perspective for therapeutic provision and practice has come from microsocial conversations among researchers, practitioners, clients themselves, and within professional bodies such as the British Association for Counselling and Psychotherapy (BACP) and user groups such as Mind. These groups share a fear that without a pluralistic perspective valuable and valid practices might be lost if they are not lost already (they may not use the word 'pluralistic', but, in effect, they argue for a more pluralistic perspective for therapy provision). The professional community of therapists and, by extension, clients who benefit from access to different modes of practice are in thrall to how monistic or pluralistic government policies and provision become. I am arguing for a broad interpretation of the word 'pluralistic'. Many practitioners make sense of their practice pluralistically even though they may never use the word 'pluralistic' and might disown Cooper and McLeod's conceptualisation of 'pluralistic therapy'.

Therapy is so much more than a sub-branch of psychology, which seems to be how many institutions and the media commonly understand it. I am 'humanistic' in its broadest meaning and particularly in my belief that therapists and therapies need to be informed by literature, films, television, theatre, comedy, music, art, and philosophy (i.e. the Humanities) as well as the narrow field of psychology: an educational background in humanities subjects, such as literature and philosophy, is perhaps a better foundation for the practice of therapy than psychology. After all, whether clients bring short stories of incidents that might have only occurred in the last week (as might interest a CBT practitioner) or long stories reaching back to infancy and childhood (as might interest psychodynamic and TA practitioners), the interpretation of stories is an art that belongs to the humanities just as much as, or more than, the discipline of psychology. The need for human beings to experience their lives as meaningful and thus prevent dysfunctional setbacks also fits into the discipline of philosophy more than psychology.

I worked as a 'mental health project worker' for several years in a 'Care in the Community' project. Although in my current practice I do occasionally see people diagnosed with 'severe and enduring mental illnesses' (SEMI), it was a particularly enlightening experience to work with that client group within the public mental health system. It allowed me to witness how people diagnosed within it can be 'treated' by those who profess to 'care'. In many ways, the projects I worked for were benign, especially within the limits of the human and financial resources available. Conversely, there was an uncritical acceptance of the medical model in which the dispensation of medications was a central task, and it seemed as if we were powerless to provide significant psychological help. The model was, at best, a biosocial one. For some residents, this could lead to a helpless acceptance of a diagnosis such as 'schizophrenia', with a contiguous belief that they could not hope for a life without their 'illness'.

One aim of the book is to explore how pluralistic approaches are impacting therapists as a whole. It appears to me that a black/white conceptualisation of pluralistic/non-pluralistic practitioners is an assumption that ultimately does not hold up. I believe all practitioners are pluralistic whether they use that word or not. It is improbable that even the most ideological and 'pure' of single-model therapists practise completely purely. At the other extreme, there is a limit to how pluralistically any therapist can realistically practise within the limits of their knowledge and experience. In that sense, I see pluralism as a dimension that runs through all therapists and therapies to greater and lesser extents, like the relationship is a dimension rather than a particular ideology or practice that must be entirely embraced or rejected. Many therapists identify to some extent with pluralistic 'values' while not identifying themselves as 'pluralistic'. For many practitioners, pluralism is not so much a 'brand' as a qualitative continuum along which practices move depending upon persons and context.

A pluralistic agenda is or might be a 'peace' agenda for the psychological therapy professions, which also relates to issues and debates about professionalisation and regulation. Therefore, engaging with how therapists might support or challenge its tenets and practices is important in understanding the ongoing struggle of the therapy profession. By embracing differences, it can present itself as a united front for its survival and progress. It is worth analysing how a pluralistic agenda is both failing and succeeding in convincing therapists that it is worthwhile.

The articulation of pluralistic therapy, from 2007 onwards, has a specific and important sociohistorical context that is elaborated upon further in the next chapter. Although there is a significant amount of 'crossover' in developments in therapy between countries, especially between the USA and the UK, the development of 'pluralism', at least as an identifying label if not a distinct idea, seems to me to be relatively localised to the UK (for instance, book sales are much higher in the UK than the USA) and has been developed in response to the UK's sociohistorical context. The trajectory from Freud in Vienna to pluralism in the UK is explored so that the phenomenon of pluralism can be contextualised within broad therapy movements such as 'integration' and narrower developments more particular to the UK, such as NHS Talking Therapies (NHSTT) and the National Institute for Health and Care Excellence (NICE).

Estimates suggest there are at least 400 different types of therapy (Kazdin, 1986), and 'critical commentators suggest the creation of so many models reflects the scientific discipline of a field in which, it seems, "anything goes"'(Feltham, 2014, p. 10). This state of affairs can be seen as 'unwieldy, confusing, and not credible' (2014, p. 10). Moreover, the assumption that different models are responsible for different levels of therapeutic effectiveness is highly questionable: 'Lambert (1992) has argued from evidence that a mere 15 per cent of client improvement is accounted for by techniques specific to designated therapy models' (2014, p. 11). (See also Bohart [2000], Cooper [2008] and Wampold [2010] for more research that supports Lambert (1992).) Nevertheless, so much research in therapy continues to ask whether therapy x is better than therapy y. These kinds of research projects ask the wrong questions and then come up with answers reflecting the initial questions' wrongness. For instance, randomised controlled trials (RCTs) are considered the 'gold standard' for therapy research by bodies such as NICE (e.g. Reeves, 2014). However, to believe in the validity of the results, one would have to assume that any given therapy acts as predictably as any medication in measured doses. Research which attempts to measure the efficacy of therapy as a kind of medicinal treatment misses the importance of the lived experience of therapists and clients in relationship to each other and in relationships external to therapy. Several MPs (UK Parliament, 2019) have challenged NICE's 'flawed methodology' (see Thornton, 2018) concerning its guidelines for depression. NICE took this seriously enough to agree to a second and even a third consultation. Both revised guidelines, however, were badly received by several stakeholder organisations, including but not limited to the Royal College of Psychiatrists (RCP), the British Psychoanalytic Council (BPC), the British Psychological Society (BPS), the Society for Psychotherapy Research (SPR), Mind, the BACP, and the UKCP (SPR, 2022; Thornton, 2018). Their responses are comprehensive and thorough, with the main agreement between these diverse organisations being that the NICE guidelines still base themselves on 'wide ranging and fundamental methodological flaws for establishing effective treatment' (Thornton, 2018). Moreover, the coalition of organisations warned that if the guidelines were published as they stood they would impede the care of millions. A major reason for this is that the organisations 'fear that a significant proportion of individuals suffering from depression could still be impeded from accessing the right treatment' (SPR, 2022). The implicit demand for a more pluralistic approach to mental health is clear.

Since the 1970s, there has been a history of moves towards integration (Feltham, 2014), but this has only added to the number of therapies on offer and has not succeeded in bridging the gaps between 'schools'. So, pluralism, as a perspective and, more arguably, as a therapeutic practice, might provide a way of embracing both singular and integrative approaches. However, even the word 'pluralism' is somewhat 'unfriendly' and unfamiliar to some therapists.

From my experience as a therapist and many conversations with therapists, I am aware of some distance between practitioners and academics/researchers, which is also reported in the literature (e.g. Norcross & Lambert, 2011b; Reeves, 2014). So, whatever the theoretical, practical and pragmatic merits of pluralistic conceptualisations of therapy may or may not be, how practising therapists experience and position themselves in relation to these ideas will ultimately be the crux on which these ideas live or die.

There are many unanswered questions about how therapists react to purist, integrative, and pluralistic conceptualisations. If 'pluralism' and 'purism' can be seen as positions, then therapists take up their positions relative to them, either practically and/or conceptually.

It is extremely difficult, if not impossible, to pinpoint what 'purism' and 'pluralism' are in the 'real world' (Robson, 2011). The words are terms that some therapists have used to construct meanings about therapy. I hope this book provides a good starting point to understand what pluralism means philosophically and politically, as well as its manifestation as 'pluralistic therapy', so that the importance of a pluralistic future for therapy from philosophical and political perspectives can inform debates about therapy and the future of therapy. I am interested in the implications of pluralism for therapeutic practice and the implications of pluralism in therapy for professional identity (Hemsley, 2013). Ultimately, I want more profound and nuanced understandings of what pluralism can mean to benefit the therapy profession and the people it serves.

Summary of the Chapters

Following this introductory chapter, the second chapter outlines a history of therapy and that history's relevance to issues of integration and pluralism within the therapy field. The manifestation of pluralism, as a useful concept for therapy in the early years of the 21st century, comes out of this long history and can only be deeply understood as a response to it. The histories of research, professionalisation, and regulation of the therapy professions are also explored as being relevant to the development of pluralism. The second chapter sets the foundation and paints the background for the subsequent chapters and their focus on the philosophical, political, and practical aspects of pluralism in relation to therapy.

Chapter 3 focuses on the philosophical meanings of pluralism; most notably for this book, on William James's conception of pluralism in his seminal *A Pluralistic Universe* (2011/1908). Other theorists such as Ken Wilber, Isaiah Berlin, Emmanuel Levinas, Andrew Samuels, Mick Cooper, and John McLeod are also discussed in relation to their understandings of pluralism and associated implications for therapy. The meanings of pluralism in relation to multiculturalism and 'cultural pluralism' are also briefly looked at before a more detailed exploration in Chapter 4, which looks at the more political meanings of pluralism.

Chapter 4 explores some of the ways pluralism has been conceptualised politically, mainly in UK and USA contexts. How these general political conceptualisations might be applied to understanding the world of therapy and its politics is also examined. In particular, the theorising of William Connolly's 'new pluralism', in which a pluralist political system is seen as more of an ideal than anything actual, is demonstrated to be relevant to thinking about therapy from a political perspective. The chapter also examines social justice and intersectionality, first discussed in Chapter 3, and how the therapy field can be understood through this lens. Centrally, the relevance of an art/science divide to pluralism is partially reflected in the embracing of or an aversion to the medical model. This also underlies issues in the politics of research.

Chapter 5 explores how therapists identify, particularly in terms of their approach or modality. It touches on the idea of superiority/inferiority complexes in the profession, a parallel to Turner's (2024) thinking about intersectionality, before exploring how professionalisation, regulation, CBT, and other issues all feed into different therapist identities.

Chapter 6 examines varying degrees of flexibility and rigidity in therapies and therapists and flexibility as a key concept in the practice of pluralistic therapy. It also explores how professionalisation and regulation impact the potential for therapists to be more or less flexible.

Chapter 7 focuses on the centrality of the relationship in therapy. I define my use of the word 'relationship' as based on Clarkson's (2003/1995) framework, which identified five different types of relationship potentially at play in any therapeutic relationship. The relational emphasis in therapy does not align well with currently privileged research methodologies and the medical model. The problems, in terms of a research-practice mismatch, are explored. Additionally, the relational aspect of different approaches, including pluralistic therapy, is compared and contrasted.

In Chapter 8, how the issues around therapist identities/approaches, flexibility, and varying emphases on the importance of the relationship led to what can be characterised as 'therapy wars' is explored. A history of the medical model and scientism in relation to therapy is outlined before exploring how pluralistic therapy might be interpreted as a kind of 'peace' agenda in reaction to these wars. Divisions over regulation, one particular war, are also discussed, as well as how research contributes to conflicts and differences within the field, particularly concerning CBT.

Chapters 9 to 11 consider how therapy theorists have proposed potential solutions to disagreements inherent in the therapy field. Chapter 9 focuses on a central concept in pluralistic therapy: metacommunication. Although this does not belong to pluralistic therapy, the practice of it undoubtedly has been emphasised in the pluralistic therapy literature more than elsewhere. It is central to pluralistic therapy's emphasis on collaboration. Metacommunication in therapy mirrors the concept of shared decision-making coming from medical practice.

Chapter 10 makes the case for tolerating uncertainty in the theory and practice of therapy rather than grasping for certainty. It then explores how uncertainty and understanding relate to modernism and postmodernism and the relationship of those concepts to pluralism and pluralistic therapy. Different views of postmodernism from pluralistic and person-centred theorists are also compared and contrasted, particularly concerning felt needs for foundational beliefs.

In Chapter 11, I examine the influence of the integrative movement, generally and with particular reference to the idea of common factors in therapy. Different therapies being conceptualised as akin to different languages, touched on in a previous chapter, is further explored in relation to integrative theory. The crucial issue of whether pluralism or integrationism are much the same thing – or have important differences – is explored and the advantages and disadvantages of conceptualising therapy in integrative and pluralistic terms are also discussed.

Chapter 12 is the concluding chapter and considers the future of therapy concerning professionalisation and regulation, generally, and with specific reference to the UK Scope of Practice and Education (SCoPEd) project and its impacts on the therapy 'landscape'. The influence of the medical model on professionalisation and regulation agendas is further explored before concluding thoughts on pluralism and pluralistic therapy and how pluralistic philosophies and politics might inform therapeutic practices. Cooper and McLeod's version of pluralistic therapy is, in particular, focussed on in terms of its impact and possibilities, as well as its more recent developments in relation to the person-centred approach (PCA). Looking towards the future, it is impossible to ignore the implications of artificial intelligence (AI) for pluralism/pluralistic therapy, as well as the potential of psychedelic therapy. Finally, I call for a more pluralistic vision for mental health services with an understanding of the philosophical and political implications of pluralism and pluralistic therapy considered throughout the book.

Chapter 2

A History of Pluralism in Therapy and Pluralistic Therapies

This chapter details how the general history of therapy, research, knowledge bases, professionalisation, and regulation link to issues of integration and pluralism in relation to therapy. There is a certain amount of crossover between different countries, particularly between the UK and the USA, but when discussing some aspects of all these issues, they are discussed with particular reference to the UK. As the book progresses, I trust that although particulars might refer more to UK and USA contexts, the importance of pluralism (generally) for therapy and therapists (generally) can be usefully compared to other national and sociohistorical contexts.

How therapeutic practices and conceptualisations of pluralism eventually come together to be named 'pluralistic therapy' at the beginning of the 21st century is a potentially vast topic, with all kinds of tangents, variables, and factors that might be argued to be important and relevant. This chapter will focus on aspects with more obvious philosophical and political implications at the micro level within the therapy field and the macro level in relation to the broader philosophical and political world. Pluralism's philosophical and political meanings will also be further explored in Chapters 3 and 4.

One of the most obvious areas in which therapy is de facto pluralistic is in the plurality and regulation of psychological practitioners. In the UK, practitioners who practise therapy, or something recognisably similar, use titles such as 'Psychological Wellbeing Practitioners' (PWPs), 'counsellors', 'psychotherapists', 'clinical psychologists', 'counselling psychologists', and 'psychiatrists'. A wide variety of educational/training levels are also required for the various titles, with initial trainings lasting anything from one to four or five years. Most practitioners, but certainly not all, also undergo various trainings after obtaining any initial qualifications, and most practitioners are required to undertake a minimum level of continuing professional development (CPD).

Amid all these professional titles, from the start, I want to be open about the fact that an implicit and sometimes explicit theme of this book is to argue the case for the importance of therapists (qualified and named as counsellors and psychotherapists) as providers of therapeutic relationships for the public. Other professional titles will be referred to solely to understand the context for those identifying specifically as counsellors and psychotherapists. In addition, therapy between one

DOI: 10.4324/9781003468332-2

therapist and one client (dyadic therapy) is the subject of concern. Although pluralism is just as important for the practice of couples therapy and family therapy, the practices are too different to necessarily fit into the arguments I am making about dyadic therapy. The implications of pluralism for those practices deserve books of their own.

Psychoanalysis, Psychotherapy, and Counselling

A fundamental point about the history of therapy is that therapy evolved in the 'modern' era (e.g. McLeod, 2013) and struggles to find a 'legitimate' place for itself in a 'postmodern' age (e.g. Polkinghorne, 1992). Postmodernism and its relationship to therapy and pluralism is discussed in more detail in Chapter 10, but, for now, the central implication of this modernist/postmodernist divide I want to draw attention to is the difference in the profession between those who wish to claim legitimacy for therapeutic practices as, for example, 'scientific' and 'evidence-based', and those who see such achievements, or even attempts to claim them, as spurious or irrelevant to the unpredictable dialogical encounters between human beings taking on identities as 'therapists' and 'clients'/'patients' (e.g. Polkinghorne, 1992; Yalom, 2015).

It is important to understand how therapy is developing in our own time through a historical lens, as it is only through that lens that we can understand how and why moves towards integration and later pluralism evolved from particular histories and how we are operating within a dialectic that is on particular trajectories with roots in what has come before. From a broad cultural perspective, various commentators have identified themes that facilitated the growth of therapy in 'Western societies', including the 'increase of individualism', 'fragmentation in [people's] sense of self', 'pressure on individuals to act rationally and control their emotions', a 'way of constructing an identity', replacing 'spiritual/religious systems [with] scientific models', and 'increasing emphasis on medical solutions to social and personal problems' (see McLeod, 2013, pp. 28–29). Some of these themes will be explored in more detail in the rest of this chapter to specifically understand the sociohistorical context of the intersection of pluralism with therapy.

Sigmund Freud, in 1886, began practising and researching what is most recognisably the root of the talking therapies practised today, including those whose proponents are most dismissive of his contributions. The fundamental basics of meeting in a particular space, at a particular time, to have a dialogue in which it is explicitly or implicitly emphasised that one partner is mostly to listen and one partner is mostly to speak was established by Freud's practice of psychoanalysis. Regarding the magnitude of influence, Freud's practice of psychoanalysis is, almost inarguably, the initial point at which contemporary therapy, in all its present pluralities, started. Freud's psychoanalysis is most easily understood as the 'original' therapy model in contextualising pluralism and its relation with therapy today.

From the beginning, therapy has been prone to splits, segments or – more positively expressed – branches. There has never been a time of unity, and even if it were argued that there was, it did not last long. From the 1900s, the plurality of therapies consisted of different branches within psychoanalysis. Freud insisted that his methods should be regarded as scientific and rational. Conversely, Jung found himself exploring a path that regarded myths, 'archetypes', and mystical experiences just as relevant, if not more so, as theories supporting therapeutic practices. These profound philosophical differences regarding the purpose and understanding of therapy as, on the one hand, a medical intervention designed to 'cure' conditions and, on the other, a more intuitive, healing practice aimed at the whole embodied and 'storied' (e.g. McAdams, 1996) person have continued to the present day. Medical versus non-medical ways of understanding therapy are significant points of difference and conflict. These are the kinds of differences that pluralistic therapy would eventually attempt to contain by emphasising that 'there can be many "right" answers' (Cooper & McLeod, 2011, p. 6).

By the 1930s, there were two major competing theoretical approaches, those broadly psychoanalytic and those broadly behavioural. Within those approaches, there were also subdivisions brought about by differing attitudes, perspectives, theories, and practices. During this time, a third approach, a 'humanistic' approach, was beginning to develop, even though it was not named as such at the time. Karen Horney, identified then and now as a 'psychoanalyst', began to challenge central tenets of Freudian theory, including 'penis envy' and a perceived over-emphasis on biological factors and childhood. Horney also suggested that other aspects of human experience needed to be understood more fully by therapists and their clients; most importantly (concerning the later development of humanistic therapies) the idea of 'self-realisation', which was a major focus of her 1950 book *Neurosis and Human Growth* (Horney, 1991/1950; see also Horney, 1937) and a term not that different to 'self-actualisation', which was first used prior to Horney's 'self-realisation' by Abraham Maslow in 1943 (Maslow, 1943).

Maslow was to become one of the innovators and figureheads of what eventually became known as 'humanistic psychology', which formed the theoretical basis for humanistic therapies and which would also be seen as the 'third force' in psychology (e.g. Maslow, 1968). Interestingly, although some might perceive humanistic psychology as in opposition to psychodynamic theories, Maslow himself saw his theory of motivation as an integration of 1) functionalism as proposed by James and John Dewey, 2) holism as proposed by Wertheimer, 3) Gestalt Psychology, and 4) even what he calls the 'dynamicism' of Freud and Adler, suggesting that humanistic psychology might be seen as a 'general dynamic' theory (Maslow, 1943). As psychology evolved into apparently different entities, enabling a pluralistic array of therapies, at least some of the branches did not dismiss or let go of previous concepts but engaged with them and sometimes integrated them into their practices. This evolution might be compared to Wilber's notion of holarchies in which evolution in theory and practice does not discard but builds upon previous manifestations to 'transcend' but also 'include' (see, e.g., Wilber, 2000).

In 1942, Carl Rogers published *Counseling and Psychotherapy* (Rogers, 1942). This work laid down the basic tenets of a non-directive therapy, at that time referred to as 'client-centred', which would take a prominent place in the array of human-istic therapies. A further split, evident in the title of Rogers's (1942) book, was the ongoing development of another profession – 'counselling'. In the USA, the Amer-ican Psychological Association (APA) founded a division in Counselling Psychol-ogy not too much later, in 1945 – although a 'counselling psychologist' might be argued to be something different to a 'counsellor' in the developing plurality of professional titles. The former title was, perhaps, a way for psychologists to claim an activity as their own that, it might be claimed, comes from social movements fo-cussed on particular areas and issues rather than a psychological model focussed on the individual (McLeod, 2013). In the UK, the BPS laid claim to both counselling and psychotherapy by forming a counselling psychology section in 1982 and es-tablishing a register for psychologists specialising in psychotherapy in 2004 (BPS, 2009). However, McLeod suggests that counselling should be seen as coming from education and voluntary organisations, in sharp contrast to the more scientifically and medically inclined psychotherapists and psychologists (McLeod, 2013).

In the same year that Rogers published the latest update of his ideas in *Client-Centered Therapy* (Rogers, 2003/1951), Gestalt therapy made its presence felt with the publication of *Gestalt Therapy* (Perls et al., 1951). Therefore, by the 1940s/1950s, the foundations of three distinct and competing approaches had been established, with humanistic therapies as the most recent addition.

In 1952, the American Personnel and Guidance Association, later to become the American Counseling Association, was founded (Leahy et al., 2015; McLeod, 2013) – the same year the Diagnostic and Statistical Manual of Mental Disor-ders (DSM) was first published. Retrospectively, it is possible to see the birth of movements with different philosophical assumptions and opposing ideas about how best to practise eventually developing into therapy cultures destined to be at odds with each other. The DSM created a common resource for the diagnosis of disorders, giving the impression of a scientific-medical certainty about hu-man experience based on symptomatology and building upon the predominantly medicalised approach of psychotherapy in this period. The model consisted of patients consulting experts who could diagnose and then offer treatments pref-erably validated by some kind of scientifically-based research. This approach contrasts significantly with the humanistic and person-centred approaches being developed during the same period. The former might be seen as more valuing of an 'instrumental' approach, while the latter humanistic and person-centred ap-proaches might be seen as more 'relational' (Rowan, 2016), although those terms had not yet been formulated.

Behavioural therapy fitted well with the medicalised, scientifically-informed approach to therapy, and throughout the 1950s, behaviourism made further pro-gress in developing therapeutic approaches. The most important contributions were made by B.F. Skinner (1953), by Albert Ellis (1955), who acknowledged the im-portance of thoughts and feelings as well as behaviour in his aptly named Rational Emotive Behavior Therapy (REBT), and Wolpe's 'reciprocal inhibition' (1958). It was also 'about the same time the medical barrier was lowered, and psychologists began to practice psychotherapy more prevalently' (Wampold & Imel, 2015, p. 20).

Although those initially trained or educated in psychology are represented in all therapeutic approaches, the particular emphasis on a more scientific sense of psychology is mainly associated with behaviourism and its associated therapeutic approaches, later to be most commonly practised as CBT. As at least part of their agenda, these kinds of therapies have the wish to promote psychotherapies closely aligned with the discipline of psychology (as opposed to philosophy, for instance). This reflects another aspect of the professional splitting and divisions around the practice of therapy, as well as disputed boundaries around who is – and who is not – thought fit to practise.

Despite these developments, humanistic therapies continued to gain influence, primarily via Maslow (1954) and Frankl (1959), the latter bringing a more existential aspect to humanistic psychology with the extremely popular and influential *Man's Search for Meaning*, much admired by Carl Rogers. The *Journal of Humanistic Psychology* was founded in 1961, and the Association of Humanistic Psychology (AHP) in 1963 (Orlans & Van Scoyoc, 2009). Also, in the 1960s, the medical model itself (elucidated further in Chapter 8 and throughout) began to be challenged more overtly by authors such as Szasz (e.g. 1960, 1961) and Laing (e.g. 1960), the latter also bringing an existential influence to bear on the practice of therapy. The Esalen Institute, founded in 1962 in Big Sur in California, was associated with humanistic psychology, especially for its use of 'encounter groups'. Carl Rogers gave lectures there, and both Fritz Perls and Gregory Bateson, leading luminaries of humanistic thought and practice, lived at Esalen for some years. It was closely allied with the 'human potential movement' (e.g. Rowan & Glouberman, 2018), and due to its association with places such as Esalen and the people who frequented such places, humanistic psychology was identified with the counter-cultural movement that took off in the mid- to late 1960s (see, for example, Grogan, 2013). This association with the 'new age' may still be an element in the conscious or perhaps unconscious marginalisation of humanistic therapies. Similarly, it might be said that this cultural/counter-cultural division is part of the ongoing 'paradigm war' in contemporary culture between a technocratic modernity and a more 'postmodern' impulse.

From Modernism to Postmodernism

If the history of therapy from the time of Freud up to the late 1970s can be characterised as the 'modern' era of therapy, from the 1980s onwards, therapy, along with other professions and cultural practices, entered the 'postmodern era'. The term 'postmodern' was used in various fields, such as the arts, and had various meanings. However, it was around this time that philosophers (e.g. Lyotard, 1984/1979) began to use it to advance a 'sceptical stance towards ... "grand narratives", or totalizing truth claims, such as Marxism, psychoanalysis, Christianity ... and their replacement by more relativistic, nuanced local knowledges' (McLeod, 2013, p. 30). This attitude towards knowledge is intertwined with pluralistic conceptualisations; in fact, some writers do not differentiate between pluralism and postmodernism (e.g. Wilber, 2000).

The philosophical foundations (or lack thereof) for a postmodern attitude towards therapy, and within the profession itself, were being laid from this time onwards and provided the context in which pluralistic philosophy would come to influence the future of the profession. Another fundamental division, in addition to the symptom/holism split, can be seen between those promulgating a more 'modern' framework for the practice of therapy and those challenging these modern conceptualisations from a postmodern perspective. The former implicitly and/ or explicitly believe in totalising, scientific, 'evidence-based' truths, such as stating one approach is definitively and inarguably better than another, while the latter postulate that therapy cannot be understood in these terms and is a practice which fundamentally does not have concrete theoretical 'foundations' of any kind (e.g. Loewenthal, 2011; Polkinghorne, 1992).

Even from a 'modern' perspective, the notion that when trying to understand the efficacy (or not) of therapy different approaches should be the variable to investigate was beginning to be dismissed, if not outside the profession, certainly from a large proportion of practitioners within it (e.g. Stiles et al., 1986). One variable posited to be more important, for instance, was that of the person of the therapist (e.g. Gilbert et al., 1989) rather than any particular technique or approach they employed.

The idea that there were all kinds of factors that might explain the effectiveness of therapy, of which the 'approach' was merely one, began to be argued by practitioners, particularly those who began to advocate for 'integrative' therapy (e.g. Norcross & Goldfried, 1992; Saltzman & Norcross, 1990). A growing interest in integrative therapy paralleled the increasing influence of postmodernism. It was marked by such events as the founding of the Society for the Exploration of Psychotherapy Integration (SEPI) in 1983 and the founding of the *Journal of Integrative and Eclectic Psychotherapy* in 1991 (Hollanders, 2014). By 2005, the political influence of psychotherapy integration on the profession was firmly established: in the second edition of the *Handbook of Psychotherapy Integration* (Norcross & Goldfried, 2005), the editors assert that 'integration has grown into a mature and international movement' (p. v). The history and context of integrative therapy and how that led to pluralistic therapy will be explored further in the last section of this chapter.

Some theorists responded to postmodern ideas directly, such as White and Epston (1990), whose 'narrative therapy' aimed, amongst other things, to externalise problems rather than locate them within the individual. This was a response to the common critique of therapy as too focussed on essentialist conceptualisations of the individual 'self' rather than upon the social structures in which the individual lives. Overall, critics sympathetic to a postmodern deconstruction of therapy problematised its practices as uncritically – and perhaps damagingly – colluding with the problems of postmodern society. Some of these critics argued that therapy provided one more way of filling the 'empty self' (e.g. Cushman, 1990) or intensified the 'social construction' of individuals being in 'deficit' rather than the postmodern society characterised by insecurities and uncertainties (e.g. Furedi, 2004; Gergen,

1990; Smail, 2005). Others were even harsher with their critiques of therapy's role in contemporary society. Masson, for example, referred to psychotherapy as being a 'tyranny' (Masson, 1992).

The philosophical, theoretical, and practical splits outlined above are the most apparent factors behind the development of pluralistic therapy. However, the influence of research practices, contestation over what the knowledge bases for therapy are and/or might be, and professionalisation and regulation are equally important. Moreover, as in other professions, the impact of an increasingly felt need to audit and monitor practice in terms of outcomes and other criteria can also be argued to set the conditions in which pluralistic approaches towards therapy might arise. These issues will be explored further in subsequent sections.

Research, Therapy, and the Randomised Controlled Trial (RCT)

The 'cases' that were Freud's first 'patients' in Vienna in 1886 could be viewed as forming the beginnings of research in therapy (e.g. Tudor, 2018a). The case study approach has continued to be used as a research method, and there have been attempts to make it more rigorous and credible. However, even within qualitative research, it still struggles to be accepted (e.g. McLeod, 2010). The association of psychotherapy with psychology (especially in the USA) (Norcross et al., 2011) and the drive for scientific credibility within psychology have fostered a culture in which quantitative research about therapy, in particular the RCT, has been taken more seriously (by both researchers and providers) than case studies and other forms of qualitative research (e.g. Tudor, 2018a).

The first randomised designs were developed in the 1920s and 1930s. They did not dominate research methodologies, however. In terms of therapy research, it was Carl Rogers who could be argued to have made the most impact in the 1940s, with his research based on transcripts of therapy sessions from audio tapes (McLeod, 2013). Rogers focussed on the process and the how, which remains an important area of therapy research but is less favoured by providers who prefer 'outcome' research. He was also interested in outcome, but not at the expense of researching process. Some generic factors are associated with positive outcomes but are not aligned with any particular approach (see, e.g., Wampold & Imel, 2015), which supports integrative and pluralistic approaches from a 'process' point of view. 'Outcome' research is effectively designed to establish winners and losers via statistical results based on 'rigorous', and consequently 'rigid', definitions and delivery of particular approaches.

The first RCT 'is typically dated to … 1948' (Bothwell & Podolsky, 2016), when the British Medical Research Council (BMRC) tested a drug 'for the treatment of tuberculosis' (2016), and the RCT is still mostly associated with attempting to determine the effectiveness of medications. In the 1950s, the 'randomized placebo control group design' was developed and has become a standard way of evaluating the efficacy of medications (Wampold & Imel, 2015). Scientific evidence was used to diminish the importance of psychotherapy when, in 1952, Eysenck 'claimed that the rate of recovery of patients receiving psychotherapy was equal to the rate of spontaneous remission' (Wampold & Imel, 2015, p. 24; Eysenck, 1952). In other words, it was claimed that therapy was not effective – quite a damaging claim for the profession and one that was widely disseminated in mainstream as well as academic media. In response to these claims, researchers attempted to increase the rigour of their studies.

Despite the severity of Eysenck's attack on psychotherapy, Wampold and Imel (2015) suggest that psychotherapy was found to be 'efficacious' by a 'meta-analysis of psychotherapy outcome studies'. Although meta-analyses of therapy were themselves a focus of Eysenck's critique, by this time, meta-analysis was the 'standard method of aggregating research results in education, psychology, and medicine' (Wampold & Imel, 2015, p. 25), so lending strong support to the claim that psychotherapy was indeed effective.

One major problem in research about therapy, then and now, is that for an RCT to be methodologically sound unwanted variables need to be flattened or taken into account so that tentative conclusions about the trial can be made. One variable which needs to be constant for the trial to have any significance (within its paradigm) is that the 'treatment' or type of therapy needs to be the same, no matter which clinician is delivering it; otherwise, the definition of what therapy is becomes too broad to have any practical meaning. Despite the likelihood that practitioners who identify with a particular approach, especially those with more experience, will vary widely in how they practise, for the sake of a successful RCT, differences between them must be minimised or eliminated. Therefore, it became necessary to determine how a treatment might become sufficiently standardised to allow scientifically valid RCTs to be undertaken. The therapeutic approach must be 'manualised' for the research and data to be perceived as valid.

The focus on the manualisation of therapy, arguably for the sake of research, changes the nature of the observed object – in this case, therapy. Those therapies that can comply with manualisation self-evidently would be advantaged as the most favoured for research. The demand that the approach be the solitary variable meant the effacing of the individual expertise of therapists and, indeed, any factors that might lie outside anything other than the approach.

Some therapies and some therapists resist manualisation, but with the dominant rise of the RCT, it would seem that it was a foregone conclusion that manualised therapies would become the therapies perceived to be scientifically validated. Therefore, the hegemony of RCTs can lead to a monoculture of therapy provision from medically-based or medically-informed providers. This historical development of therapy research was a significant factor in practitioners gravitating towards more non-competitive, integrative models of practice, which would later lead to a pluralistic framework and approach. The human element of the practitioner needing to be effectively erased for the sake of validation seemed, for some practitioners and many researchers, a step too far. Other ways of evaluating therapy from more integrative and pluralistic standpoints began to be called for by those who problematised RCTs as an ineffective research model for both process- and outcome-based research.

Overall, the drive was towards standardisations of therapies and standardisations of 'disorders' for research to have more validity within medical models of practice. Standardisation is achieved by controlling for the variables of the therapist, the client, and the presenting symptoms to ensure that the only variable being measured is the effectiveness of a particular approach. RCTs, therefore, are also problematic because what is being measured becomes something which, it might be argued, is not recognisable as what most therapists and most clients have experienced as therapy (e.g. Wampold & Imel, 2015). However, within medical systems, general functions of therapy, such as examining the unexamined life (Plato/Tredennick & Tarrant, 2003/1954), are considered too vague to be 'medical'. Therefore, research about therapeutic approaches so that they might gain influence within medical establishments needed to demonstrate that they could treat specific 'disorders' via 'clinical' trials to 'establish the viability of particular treatments for particular disorders' (Wampold & Imel, 2015, p. 24).

It could be said that the practice of research about therapy became akin to the tail wagging the dog, in the sense that therapeutic practice, at least in a research context, was being led by what research required it to be rather than research being required to adapt to the idiosyncrasies of therapeutic practice. Therapeutic practice within the RCT method is viewed in the same way as medications for physical diseases. The assumption is that the therapist is much like a doctor treating a mental 'disease', so the RCT methodology is not seen as problematic. Although some argue that research is important for practitioners to learn from, this particular kind of research led to a 'gap' between those who researched therapy and those who practised it. For some, it felt irrelevant to their practice (e.g. Talley et al., 1994).

NICE and other governmental and organisational developments will be explored in subsequent sections. For now, the main point to note is that the way research about therapy developed, with increasing emphasis on medical and scientific credibility, led to increasing alienation between practitioners, researchers, and providers (e.g. Dattilio et al., 2010).

The Knowledge Bases of Therapy

McLeod (2013) argues that therapy has a 'long-standing tradition' of being an 'interdisciplinary activity' (p. 43) while suggesting that it is also perceived increasingly as a branch of psychology. He suggests that the 'use of the term "psychological therapies" and the expansion of counselling psychology have reinforced this trend' (p. 43). He argues that other disciplines, such as philosophy and neuroscience, are important knowledge bases for therapy. Rabu and McLeod (2018) similarly argue that therapy 'draws on multiple sources of knowledge, including personal knowledge ... theoretical knowledge ... and scientific knowledge' (p. 776).

Psychology is a major foundation for diverse therapies, and unsurprisingly a multiplicity of therapeutic approaches reflects the multiplicity of psychological theories. Often, no distinctions are made between psychology and therapy, which has implications for claims of distinct and clear knowledge bases for different therapies, no matter the psychological approach upon which they draw.

From a philosophical perspective, different therapeutic theories might be perceived to reflect different worldviews, and some research supports the idea that therapists are attracted to different therapeutic approaches based on their philosophical positions (e.g. Lyddon & Bradford, 1995).

Neuroscience is becoming increasingly important for the knowledge bases of therapy, and many theoreticians argue that therapists should at least have a basic understanding of the subject (e.g. Montgomery, 2013). While important advances have been made, the relevance of these findings to understanding human experience in its idiosyncratic contexts is arguable, and some renounce the enthusiasm for neuroscience in the fields of psychology and therapy as a contemporary 'neuromania' (see Tallis, 2011).

McLeod (2013) asserts that '[a]ttempts to fuse counselling and psychotherapy into a single *psychological* therapy will never be successful' (p. 53, emphasis in original) because, he argues, the influence of multiple disciplines on therapy is too important for its practices to be only located within psychology. However, because from an academic perspective singular disciplines are more powerful, and the discipline of psychology is particularly powerful, there has been a tendency for trainings to locate therapy within it. Pluralism and pluralistic therapy directly challenge this tendency towards wanting to integrate counselling and psychotherapy within psychology. This may be theoretically responsible, but professionally and academically it is disadvantageous. The philosophical basis of pluralistic therapy faces challenges on this pragmatic front.

However, a pluralistic understanding of therapy has the potential to include all the potential knowledge bases of therapy in education and training. This pluralistic perspective would not obligate educators and trainers to provide training/education in everything. However, it would emphasise that trainings – 'counselling' or 'psychotherapy' at postgraduate, masters, or doctoral levels – are merely introductions into a practice which relies primarily on experience and continuous, open-ended learning (McLeod et al., 2016). This may go against instrumental notions demanding that trainees know everything they need to know before being seen as 'qualified', but it is probably a more realistic view of what happens in practice. Many therapists are uncertain about their abilities in the early days of being officially qualified: for some, this uncertainty remains and yet others come to the view that – paradoxically – living with uncertainty and being comfortable with 'not knowing' is a central qualification of being a competent therapist.

McLeod (2013) argues that psychotherapists base their practice on one approach, whereas counsellors draw on different approaches depending on 'their relevance to a particular client or group' (p. 58). He is making the case for counselling as pluralistic. This attempt to distinguish counselling and psychotherapy by suggesting the former to be more pluralistic is, arguably, a misguided attempt to find a unique jurisdiction for 'counselling' that is unnecessary and undermines the personal and professional potential of all therapists, including 'counsellors'.

Therefore, counselling and psychotherapy have similar and overlapping knowledge bases, and issues about pluralism apply to one as much as the other. I hold this view while acknowledging that wanting to distinguish counselling from psychotherapy does respect a pluralistic position.

From this perspective, both counselling and psychotherapy, or 'therapy', can be seen to have evolved a multiplicity of approaches by developing distinct theories, languages, practices, 'knowledge communities', values, and mythologies (McLeod, 2013).

McLeod (2013) suggests that the multiplicity of approaches and the debates they foster may be less about actual differences and more about what languages are best to articulate practice – the idea many therapists share that often supposedly different approaches have 'different names for the same thing'. Understanding different therapeutic approaches as akin to different languages will be explored further in Chapter 11.

McLeod (2013) further asserts that the manifestation of these various approaches reflects everyday commercial interests in establishing 'brand name therapies' (see also Gopaldas, 2016 on therapy as a 'marketplace icon'), which are selling more or less the same thing (despite his insistence that there are real differences between counselling and psychotherapy).

Schwarz (1955 cited in O'Connell, 2005) identifies 'three stages through which new theories pass' (p. 8), which consist of, first, the 'Essentialist' stage in which 'competing schools … [claim] superiority' (p. 8), secondly, the 'Transitional', in which 'followers themselves begin to recognise limitations to their model' (p. 8), and thirdly, the 'Ecological', which is a 'process of integrating with other ideas, accompanied by an understanding of the constantly evolving nature of the field. In this stage, a more eclectic position may emerge' (p. 8). Therapy – in a 'holarchical' (e.g. Wilber, 2000) way, which views evolution as transcending yet including what has come before – seems currently to reflect all three stages. The first stage is encouraged by a research culture that wants answers to what schools are superior; the second and third stages might be seen as reflecting integrative and, more recently, pluralistic movements in the field.

Whether or not different therapeutic approaches describe the same phenomena, they all lay claim to a specialist body of theory and knowledge, and it is these theories and knowledge bases that fundamentally allow therapists to claim to be 'professionals'. A distinguishing feature of a 'professional project' (see Larson, 1977) is that there is a recognisable knowledge base, the use of which should be restricted to the recognised members of the profession (Waller, 2009). However, the multidisciplinary nature of therapy challenges the articulation of a consensual knowledge base. In other words, the pluralism of knowledge bases for the practice of therapy, which some would suggest includes not just a multitude of psychological theories but also different philosophies and the humanities, has led to differences of opinion as to what precisely constitutes the knowledge bases of therapy.

The literature suggests that the factors of effective therapy, sometimes at least, do not go much further than the client, the therapist, and the relationship they create between them. In other words, the very need for knowledge bases for the practice of therapy is debatable, and if that is contestable, then so is the view of therapy as a profession. If therapy is an activity in which 'personality' is more important than 'theory', then the standard criteria for professionalisation are difficult to apply (Waller, 2009). Nevertheless, despite these difficulties, the professionalisation of therapy (both 'counselling' and 'psychotherapy') continues unabated, and this process of professionalisation (premised on educational criteria) will be further explored in subsequent sections.

Professionalisation, Regulation, Audit Culture, Managed Care, and Evidence-Based Medicine

Therapy and the Sociology of the Professions

Counselling and psychotherapy can be viewed as being in the midst of a 'professional project' (e.g. Larson, 1977), which, in the UK particularly, has been beset by problems. Pressure groups, such as the Alliance for Counselling and Psychotherapy (ACP) (originally called the Alliance for Counselling and Psychotherapy Against State Regulation), actively campaigned against SR, resisting the furtherance of the project, which was simultaneously supported more keenly (although still with some ambiguity) by therapy's professional or 'occupational' associations such as the BACP and the UKCP. Macdonald suggests that a 'feature of the professional project is the internecine strife that occurs in the early stages, as different occupational strands or professional philosophies contend for power' (Macdonald, 1995, p. 138). Pluralism, in this sense, can be seen as related to professionalisation and regulation and reflecting the 'internecine strife' of the therapy field as it engages in a professional project to achieve social closure, market control, status, and respectability (e.g. Macdonald, 1995). Macdonald (1995) asserts that in the '[state/profession relationship] ... conflicts tend to get resolved in the long run' (p. 119). Whether this turns out to be the case for counselling, psychotherapy, and whatever other names might be applied to therapeutic activities remains to be seen. The intangible nature of the meaning of 'therapy' and the multiple divisions of opinion about its meaning might have produced a knot too tricky to untangle. This is in addition to the issue of differentiating counsellors, psychotherapists, clinical psychologists, mental health nurses, and other allied professionals who practise therapy. Many professionals claim they can, and indeed do, practise therapy but do not bear the titles of either 'counsellor' or 'psychotherapist'. Macdonald (1995) refers to the 'Marxian sociology of the professions' (p. 22), which as well as highlighting the relationship of professionalisation to the state also observes the 'proletarianization of professional occupations' (p. 22), especially one might add when they have not achieved social closure. The practice of therapy by allied professionals such as nurses and the newly titled 'Psychological Wellbeing Practitioners' (PWPs) exemplifies a profession that has failed to accomplish 'social closure' (e.g. de Swaan, 1990). Similarly, a weakness in the professionalisation of CBT is the perception of it as a collection of techniques (which, therefore, might not need a specific kind of professional to deliver them) as opposed to a highly skilled activity because 'association of technique with knowledge is one of the potential weak points in the professional armour, for if the technique can be separated from knowledge then the door is opened for other occupations to encroach' (Macdonald, 1995, p. 184).

Concerning the conflict between 'counselling' and 'psychotherapy', it has failed to achieve 'dual closure', which is when 'occupations ... having been successfully excluded by an occupation, strive to carve out their own occupational field, distinguishing it from that of other, probably dominant groups but establishing at the same time their own exclusionary practices' (1995, p. 133). This is problematic in the counselling/psychotherapy divide because some psychotherapists, especially in the private sector, would be disadvantaged by being unable to offer 'counselling', and it is arguable that counsellors do not offer 'psychotherapy' – so the jurisdiction of both activities (if, in fact, they do differ) is often claimed by counsellors and psychotherapists.

In the sociology of the professions, it is recognised that 'problems ... confront many occupations pursuing their professional project' (Macdonald, 1995, p. 140) because it is difficult to '[define] themselves, their work, their jurisdiction and their market in a way that will satisfy all interested parties' (p. 140); and further, 'professional unity is necessary if a professional body is to be sufficiently impressive to obtain state recognition' (1995, p. 199). These insights foreshadow the problems which attempts to professionalise therapy have encountered. These problems and other issues are explored in the next section, which will provide an overview of the professionalisation and regulation of therapy.

The Professionalisation and Regulation of Therapy

In 1999, Lord John Alderdice brought together stakeholder groups to statutorily regulate 'psychotherapy' but not 'counselling'. The BAC (as it was then) was unhappy about being excluded, and Alderdice remembered saying: 'I'm not talking about regulating what you are describing and if there are any of your people who are psychotherapists of course they would be able to be regulated' (Alderdice, 2009 in Aldridge, 2011). This statement demonstrates a surprising lack of knowledge and confusion from someone nominally directing the regulation of psychological therapies. Even if the only point of consensus is that both psychotherapists and counsellors talk to people in confidence, if one profession was felt to require regulation, then that would imply regulation of the other, as a major stated aim of regulation is to 'protect' the public. If psychotherapists alone were regulated, then unscrupulous or regulation-averse practitioners would merely have to change their title from 'psychotherapist' to 'counsellor' to enter an unregulated profession. Again, this confusion about 'counselling' and 'psychotherapy' and whether one is more 'professional' (and therefore more worthy of regulation) remains unresolved.

As Aldridge wittily put it in her research journal: 'It seems that there is now a direct confrontation facing us between the evidence that finds no difference between counselling and psychotherapy and the political view, that there is a difference even if we don't know what it is' (Aldridge, 2011, p. 390). In any case, the government rejected Alderdice's private members' bill attempting to regulate psychotherapy in 2001.

It was only in 2007, with the publication of the White Paper 'Trust, Assurance and Safety – The Regulation of Health Professionals in the 21st Century' (e.g. Department of Health, 2007; see, for example, HCPC, 2017), which proposed that counselling and psychotherapy be regulated by the Health Professions Council (HPC), that the potential reality of SR began to gain momentum. On the recommendation of this paper, in the same year, the HPC 'announced [their] intention to investigate and make recommendations to the Secretary of State for Health on the statutory regulation of counsellors and psychotherapists' (Lawton & Nash, 2013, p. 44) and duly formed a Professional Liaison Group (PLG) to help them in this aim.

The UKCP, from the late 1980s onwards, established a section known as the 'Humanistic and Integrative Section' (HIPS) to include humanistic and integrative therapies. It is notable that the Department of Health (DH), when setting out a 'modality training list for psychotherapy', excluded 'Humanistic and Integrative Psychotherapy from this list' (Lawton & Nash, 2013, p. 44.) at about the same time as it was inviting the HPC to consider the possibility of regulating counselling and psychotherapy. Even though this was claimed to be a 'mistake', at least from a Freudian point of view, it is an interesting one. At the first fence, Skills for Health (a not-for-profit organisation influential in the NHS for ideas on how to improve the workforce) had failed to acknowledge the potential importance of a pluralistic perspective for regulation. The impression of organisations representing humanistic and integrative therapies was that there was an attempt to marginalise them, and many individuals and organisations campaigned for humanistic and integrative therapies to be included.

Nevertheless, in 2008, Skills for Health excluded humanistic and integrative modalities, claiming that 'other modalities are variants of [psychoanalytical/psychodynamic, cognitive behavioural, and family/systemic]'. The Prime Minister's Office stated that '[w]e wish to avoid an increase in different types, or modalities, of psychotherapy' (cited in Lawton & Nash, 2013, p. 46). Eventually, the Prime Minister's Office retracted its initial statement that regulation would be restricted to only three modalities. However, these events illustrate a wish to simplify the plurality of psychological therapies from hundreds of approaches (e.g. Orlans & Van Scoyoc, 2009) to, in that instance, just three. Those who wish to professionalise and regulate have a simultaneous interest in homogenisation and standardisation so that standards and rules can be more efficiently designed. On this basis alone, there is resistance to a pluralistic agenda.

There is an intense desire, however, for the perceived professional status of being regulated, so the UKCP HIPS section eventually agreed that they would refer to themselves as '"Humanistic Integrative" or "Integrative Humanistic"'(Lawton & Nash, 2013, p. 46) as if the two related but distinct meanings could merge without controversy. Although some theoreticians perceive integrative therapy as existing within a humanistic umbrella (e.g. Gilbert & Orlans, 2011), it is possible to be humanistic but not integrative and integrative but not humanistic. Definitions and distinctions were fudged in the hope of achieving regulated status, demonstrating how practitioners and regulators can misunderstand and deceive each other for their own ends. In relation to pluralism and therapy, specifically, it might be argued that because the PLG did not support regulating specific modalities, it was supportive of a pluralistic agenda. However, in general, common misunderstandings, such as failing to differentiate between humanistic and integrative therapeutic approaches, indicate the challenge to recognise, celebrate, and tolerate differences central to a pluralistic agenda.

The HPC published its report 'Consultation on the statutory regulation of psychotherapists and counsellors' in 2009 (HPC, 2009). Regarding pluralism, the BACP (2009) agreed with the PLG's recommendation to the HPC that the regulation of approaches was too problematic. The most controversial aspect of the report was how the PLG wanted to differentiate between counsellors and psychotherapists. There are various complaints in the BACP response to the HPC report. However, it mostly elaborates on their insistence that there should be no differentiation between counselling and psychotherapy and, therefore, no differentiation between counsellors and psychotherapists. Although they do agree with both professions' titles being protected, the argument that there is no distinction between counselling and psychotherapy yet agreement that there should be two separate and different titles for practitioners of the same activity (rather than one title such as 'psychological therapist') seems contradictory. In relation to pluralism, attempts to erase difference between counselling and psychotherapy might be seen as an attempt at integration, whereas to try to tease out differences respects a more pluralistic position.

Although the BACP, for a long time, did not recognise any difference between counselling and psychotherapy, some practitioners do perceive differences. Some counsellors would like to claim jurisdiction over some practices, such as basing themselves in community-based projects rather than health centres (e.g. McLeod, 2013), and some psychotherapists would like to claim jurisdiction over other practices, such as working at a 'deeper ... level ... over a longer period, usually with more disturbed clients' (2003, p. 11). Both claims are highly arguable, and even McLeod, who favours making distinctions, suggests that these differences, amongst several he identifies, be seen as a 'direction of travel' rather than a 'fixed map' (p. 13).

Managed Care

The concept of 'managed mental health care' refers to the attempt to manage costs within healthcare systems (e.g. Bento, 2016). Therapies seen as cost-effective and

efficient have inevitably come to dominate provision, to the extent that there is little if any choice of therapeutic approach or practice for clients seeking their health
care via organisations such as the NHS. This puts pressure on therapists and the
proponents of the therapeutic approaches they use to demonstrate efficiencies of
practice that were not traditionally part of the psychotherapeutic agenda. For some
therapists, the reduction of a Generalised Anxiety Disorder (GAD) score is enough
and proves efficiency; for others, it merely scratches the surface of a broader self-
narrative in which it is possible, for example, that even a reduced score might
actually be reflective of learning how to bury a problem rather than cope with it.
The principles of managed health care, which inform how large organisations such
as the NHS and some Employee Assistance Programmes (EAPs) conceptualise
therapy provision, have profound implications for the provision of pluralistic perspectives and practices.

The most apparent effect of the growing influence of managed care policies was
the drift of therapeutic provision to the briefest forms of therapy and also those that
could claim 'evidence-based' status. This would lead to a narrowing of choice for
therapists and clients concerning how they could conform to providers' expectations. This narrowing of choice would also set the ground from which a call for a
more pluralistic approach might become more vocal and challenging of the existing order.

At philosophical and ethical levels, therapists have also been obligated to accept conceptualising therapy as part of a larger 'kind of medical consumerism'
(Cushman & Gilford, 1999). The ideologies of managed care could not help but
influence how therapists practise, and its implicit assumptions seep into the therapeutic relationship. Cushman and Gilford (1999) suggest that: '[d]espite consumer
satisfaction-like questionnaires and post-test measures, the overall power relation
of expert to object seems to continue unabated … in the social terrain of managed
care, patients come to light as objects of technicist intervention' (p. 25).

Further, Cushman and Gilford (1999) suggest that managed care, in its impact on
the practice of therapy, reflects a culture in which 'everyday survival strategies ne-
cessitate a life devoid of a deep self with a complex – and singular – subjectivity',
since such a self is 'conterminous with the intensified valorization of speed, efficiency, and productivity' (p. 27). In this culture, the 'concerns of labor are erased
by an unquestioned acceptance of management's profit motive' (p. 28). In the way
that practices reflect the wider cultures around them, this would apply not just to
workers locating their problems within themselves and their perceived inability
to cope with environmental pressures (rather than unreasonable demands by em-
ployers, perhaps) but also to therapists submitting to, or uncritically accepting, the
demand that their practices should prioritise efficiency over effectiveness.

In the UK, the growth of managed care in its health systems began with the introduction of free market ideology in the 1980s (Lees, 2016) and the ideas of the
New Public Management (NPM) (Ferlie et al., 1996). For managers to make the
best decisions, however, they needed evidence – hence the importance of evidence-
based medicine and, consequently, evidence-based therapies.

Evidence-Based Medicine, Evidence-Based Practice, NICE, IAPT, and CBT

Evidence-based medicine can be conceptualised as a three-legged stool in which 'the use of evidence (first leg) is to be balanced with the expertise of the clinician (second leg) and characteristics and context of the patient (third leg)' (Wampold & Imel, 2015, p. 11). It has been further described as making 'use of individual patients'… preferences in making clinical decisions about their care' (Sackett et al., 1996, p. 71). Sackett et al. (1996) warn that 'without clinical expertise, practice risks becoming tyrannised by evidence, for even excellent external evidence may be inapplicable to or inappropriate for an individual patient' (p. 72). It is important to note that in these conceptualisations of evidence-based medicine, which are mainly sympathetic and uncritical, evidence is not seen as superior to 'clinical expertise', and in relation to pluralistic approaches to therapy, it is also not seen as superior to patient choice. However, arguably, in the practical application of evidence-based medicine, it seems as if two legs of the stool have been taken away, with just the first leg (that of evidence) being considered, with the wishes of clinicians and patients being demoted if not forgotten. This was how some practitioners viewed the impact of evidence-based medicine in the USA. It is also how many practitioners began to view it in the UK, especially since the establishment of the National Institute for Clinical Excellence (NICE) in 1999 (its title was later changed to the National Institute for Health and Care Excellence, but it uses the same abbreviation).

Therefore, in the sociohistorical developments of the therapy profession in the UK, a trajectory can be traced from competing interests within the profession itself, leading to an emphasis on research which then leads to an emphasis on the RCT. In response to the context of a developing audit culture and that culture's need for evidence and efficiency, CBT, with its evidence base and perceived efficiency, then comes to dominate the provision of therapy, and other approaches lose their status and are marginalised, if not erased, from public providers. The private sector continued to provide employment opportunities for practitioners of other approaches (and this issue will be explored in other chapters), but within the NHS, CBT, to a great extent, began to monopolise therapy provision. It is the same in the USA, where 'multiple surveys have shown that licensed practitioners in the public systems tend to be more CBT and short-term, whereas those in private practice more psychodynamic, humanistic and the like' (Norcross, 2023).

In 2008, adding to the plurality of psychological practitioners, the DH produced an implementation plan for the training of 'low-intensity therapies workers' who would facilitate the use of CBT via 'guided self-help and computerised CBT' (Department of Health, 2008, p. 3). These workers would become known as 'Psychological Wellbeing Practitioners' (PWPs) and be perceived as fit to practise after 45 days of training (p. 3). One advantage, in terms of cost, is that these practitioners could expect a maximum pay rate less than even a trainee psychotherapist. Therefore, therapists in the NHS were not only coming under pressure in terms of their approaches being devalued but also in terms of their professional opportunities being 'undercut' by the creation of jobs/titles purportedly needing less expertise, a 'proletarianisation' of therapeutic practice.

It is against this background of an audit culture which based its decisions about therapy provision on narrow definitions of evidence that led from a pluralistic perspective to the monistic hegemony of CBT. The pluralistic framework of Cooper and McLeod (2007; 2011) can be interpreted as an evolutionary or dialectical response to these developments. It might also be interpreted as a response specific to the UK (its influence seems not to have impacted the USA significantly), as a way of presenting therapeutic practices to UK stakeholders in a comprehensible manner, using a new term that was not as tired or as researched as 'integrative'. The focus of the next section will be how integrative therapy came to develop or engender pluralistic therapy and what, if any, differences there are between the two approaches.

Integrative Therapy to Pluralistic Therapy

Watson (1940) suggested that there were 'areas of agreement in psychotherapy' such as a common belief in the importance of the therapeutic relationship. He also made another important point: 'agreement is greater in practice than in theory' (p. 708). Similar to the research/practice gap, this reflects that there is also a theoretical approach/practice gap. In other words, how practitioners practise does not necessarily align with the principles of their identified approaches (e.g. Spurling, 2016). Some practitioners pay barely any attention to the theoretical principles of different approaches, except in the most cursory sense, and this view has been supported and theorised in different ways by academics and researchers (e.g. Loewenthal, 2011).

Lazarus (1967) 'introduced the concept of technical eclecticism', which proposed 'using therapy methods advocated by different orientations without having to accept the theoretical underpinning of those orientations' (Goldfried et al., 2011, p. 273). A few years later, he formalised his ideas with a distinct approach called 'multimodal therapy' (Lazarus, 1970). The pragmatic nature of this attitude to practice would later be reflected in the pluralistic approach.

Wilber's (1979) *No Boundary* focussed on how Western therapeutic approaches might be compared to and contrasted with Eastern spiritual practices and how specific therapeutic approaches might be more or less useful for specific stages of development. Although he has generally not been acknowledged by mainstream practitioners and researchers, Wilber points to the integration of meditative practices into therapy. One example of such integration is what CBT practitioners in the 2000s termed 'third wave' CBT, consisting primarily of a generic Mindfulness-Based Cognitive Therapy (MBCT) programme. These practitioners did not acknowledge Wilber's influence, but his influence is acknowledged more openly by those identifying overtly as 'transpersonal' psychologists or therapists, especially in the USA. In the UK, the late John Rowan was the leading exponent of Wilber's ideas (e.g. Rowan, 2016), but Wilber's influence on therapy in the UK is not wide-spread. Nevertheless, the idea that different therapies might be helpful for different stages of personal development has parallels with what the pluralistic approach would be arguing some years later.

Gilbert and Orlans (2011) suggest there are four definitions of integration which may or may not overlap with each other in any given integrative approach: 1) a 'holistic view of the person ... as an integrated whole', 2) the 'integration of theories and/or concepts and/or techniques', 3) the 'integration of the personal and the professional' and 4) the 'integration of research and practice' (pp. 22–23). Other ways of integrating therapies include '[a]ssimilative integration', '[h]olistic integration', '[d]isorder-specific or problem-oriented integration', '[m]ulticultural and culturally adapted therapy', 'feminist therapy', and 'collective integration' (McLeod & Sundet, 2016, pp. 159–160).

In the early 1990s, postmodernists such as Polkinghorne (1992), discussed in a previous section, were also making strong theoretical statements challenging the claim that any one theory could claim precedence over any other while simultane-ously arguing for the acceptance that the experience of actual practice, by indi-vidual therapists with individual clients in particular contexts, was more important than theoretical constructs. In postmodernist terms that elude modernist certainties, Polkinghorne argued that:

> therapists use previously effective actions as a guide for their future actions; their clinical experiences are the source of their knowledge. Yet experience is not seen as a foundation for sure knowledge. Experience itself is the repository of previous constructions.
>
> (Polkinghorne, 1992, p. 158)

Polkinghorne further suggests that '[s]uccessful therapy has been accomplished by therapists committed to various conceptual networks and practicing a variety of techniques. The psychology of practice accepts the concept of equifinality – that the same result can be achieved through a variety of approaches' (1992, p. 161). The neopragmatic, postmodern sensibility of these kinds of arguments reflects al-most exactly what Cooper and McLeod (2007), who acknowledge postmodernism as a significant influence on their pluralistic approach, will be saying in the first decade of this century.

Petruska Clarkson (2003/1995) also wrote with a sensibility influenced by postmodernism. Clarkson conceptualised an integrative framework based on five different types of therapeutic relationship, which she suggested 'are potentially present in any psychotherapeutic encounter' (p. xii). This model was influential enough to form the basis of some integrative trainings in the UK and helped ad-vance the cause of integrative therapy more generally.

The literature supporting an integrative view from theoretical, research-driven, and practitioner perspectives expanded throughout the 1990s (e.g. Hubble et al., 1999; Miller et al., 1997) in the UK and the USA. There was a certain amount of mutual support and influence between the two countries around integrative therapy, but it is noticeable in the literature that there is not as much exchange as might be expected between practitioners and researchers sharing the same language, if not the same country.

The contexts of provision vary widely between the USA and the UK: in the former, a culture exists in which health costs are funded mainly by health insurance and, in terms of providing therapy, a culture in which, for the most part, psychologists and social workers have pushed for their professions to be the licensed providers of therapy. In the UK, in the context of the NHS, although clinical psychologists have been successful in staking their claims of expertise, the separate and differentiated trainings of counsellors and psychotherapists have been clearer in terms of recognition and professionalisation. In other words, the notion of counsellors and psychotherapists as differentiated professions with different skill sets from psychologists and other 'psy professionals' (e.g. Walker et al., 2015) has been established more successfully. In the USA, from the literature (e.g. Norcross et al., 2011), it often seems that psychotherapy is viewed as a practice that belongs to an array of practitioners, from social workers to psychiatrists, but especially psychologists, whereas in the UK, the idea that psychotherapy belongs to psychotherapists and counselling belongs to counsellors seems relatively more embedded. Space precludes a further exploration of this issue here, but in contextualising integration and pluralism in the UK, it needs to be borne in mind. As argued earlier, pluralistic therapy might be seen as a particularly 'local' version of American integrative therapy, responding to local circumstances more effectively than might be afforded by identifying with the older, more established integrative movement.

Practitioners themselves responded positively to integrative ideas. Hollanders and McLeod (1999) surveyed over 300 British therapists and found that '49 per cent ... reported themselves as *explicitly* eclectic/integrative, with another 38 per cent being *implicitly* eclectic/integrative (identifying themselves with a single theoretical model but also acknowledging being influenced by other models)' (McLeod, 2013, p. 362, italics in original). The large number of therapists who identify with single approaches but actually derive their practice from more than one approach supports the contention that there is a gap between espoused theories (how therapists think they practise) and how they actually practise.

These kinds of theory–practice–research gaps are problematic for the therapy profession, as '[o]n the one hand most practice guidelines and research, and many training courses, are organised after single-model lines. On the other hand, the majority of practitioners describe themselves as deploying some kind of combination of approaches' (McLeod & Sundet, 2016, p. 159; Norcross et al., 2005; Thoma & Cecero, 2009). Unsurprisingly, organisations responsible for providing therapy understand it as a competition between single models, since this is how the therapy profession has historically presented itself, even though many practitioners are not actually wedded to single models. The integrative movement and, latterly, the pluralistic approach have attempted to transform the conceptualisation of therapy, and although they may have won over therapists themselves (to some extent), they certainly have not, on the whole, won over the institutions and organisations within which they practise.

Cooper and McLeod suggest that their 'pluralistic framework for counselling and psychotherapy' (2007) is a development that differentiates itself from integrative and eclectic positions because '[integrative and eclectic positions] have not been successful in generating research and have resulted in a further proliferation of competing models' (p. 135). They also suggest that their pluralistic approach operates as a metatheoretical model rather than as a theoretical model in itself. Nevertheless, the idea that therapy can be conceptualised to work at different levels of abstraction (technical, strategic, and theoretical) has been part of therapeutic literature and practice for many years (e.g. Wampold & Imel, 2015). In particular, the conception of metatheoretical positions could be argued to go back as far as Wilber (1979), and by the time Cooper and McLeod (2007) suggested their pluralistic framework, there actually existed a host of metatheoretical conceptualisations about therapy. Therefore, we are faced with the paradox that metatheories, at least partly designed to transcend competition between theoretical models, have created further competition at a different level.

However, a metatheoretical framework had not, perhaps, been articulated so well in the UK. Cooper and McLeod (2007) seem particularly concerned about the consequences of the lack of pluralistic theory and practice, especially regarding training, NICE guidelines and therapy provision within the NHS. This reflects a local agenda and supports the notion that the creation of pluralistic therapy, as a way of understanding and practising therapy, had specific ambitions within the UK. The subtitle of their 2007 paper is 'implications for research', which also reflects their ambition that their conceptualisation should create evidence that will change the provision and practice of therapy (in the UK, particularly). The use of the word 'pluralism' (and the underlying philosophies associated with pluralism) also suggests a postmodernist perspective more overtly than the titling of other theoretical or metatheoretical models. In some ways, this is a brave move, but in other ways, it could be seen as an obstacle to therapists with a less philosophical attitude, who might be discouraged from using the ideas for their own practice or research. There is an additional problem with the oxymoronic notion of a singular 'pluralistic therapy'. This might be less problematic if Cooper and McLeod did not suggest relatively comprehensive protocols for practising pluralistic therapy in relation to goals, tasks, and methods.

In terms of differentiating integration from pluralism, by the time Cooper and McLeod published their book on pluralistic therapy (Cooper & McLeod, 2011), they were still attempting to differentiate it on the grounds of having philosophical and ethical, rather than psychological, bases and their emphasis on collaboration with the client. However, at least some integrative therapists would also articulate integrative therapy as having a philosophical base and valuing collaboration (e.g. Gilbert & Orlans, 2011; Miller et al., 2005). Therefore, it is perhaps not surprising that there is an admission that '[p]luralistic therapy is an integrative approach' (Cooper & McLeod, 2011, p. 6). In later publications, pluralistic therapy is described as a '"collaborative integrative" way of working' (Cooper, 2015, p. 4), a 'meta-integrative framework' (McLeod & Sundet, 2016, p. 158), and a 'radical eclectic approach' (2016, p. 167) – phrases that seem to struggle to encapsulate substantial differences to integrative and eclectic approaches.

These issues about whether pluralistic therapy can claim to be anything different from what has come before will be raised and elaborated further in subsequent chapters of this book. Also, looking forward, it will be argued that if pluralism can be understood more deeply and precisely in terms of its philosophical and political meanings, then pluralism can be a prism through which all therapies and therapists can be viewed. This could lead to an evolutionary step forward for therapy in terms of a more appropriate philosophical basis (as opposed to a medical or scientific one) for theory, practice, and research and a more politically-informed basis for understanding how the therapy professions might act both for themselves and the public. These themes will be explored further as the book progresses.

Concluding Thoughts

This chapter has demonstrated how the history of psychoanalysis, psychotherapy, and counselling has led to research methodologies which fit in with – and encourage the acceptance of – audit cultures, managed care, and evidence-based practice in what might be succinctly described as the postmodern, neoliberal era from the late 1980s onwards. The professionalisation and regulation of therapy run alongside these developments, and all these issues have caused, and continue to cause, divisions among practitioners. Integrationism in therapy, on one level, might be seen as a reaction to modernist views on the practice of psychotherapy – views which led to a 'winner-takes-all' attitude to different therapeutic approaches. The belief that different therapies can be measured and validated efficiently – and unproblematically – alongside the construction of specific forms of quantitative research (i.e. RCTs) has threatened the evolution of a dynamic, pluralistic therapy culture.

The therapy professions still appear to be greatly confused about the theories that drive their practices. This confusion has led to disagreements and then attempts to create a more inclusive way of conceptualising practice (i.e. integration/pluralism). However, some practitioners remain sympathetic to a 'modern' sense of quasi-certainty, allowing some therapeutic approaches to be seen as definitively better than others. Unquestionably, there are advantages and disadvantages for different types of practitioners holding onto modern or postmodern conceptualisations of therapy. These differences reflect extant 'therapy wars' (Saltzman & Norcross, 1990). These therapy wars are referred to in more detail in Chapter 8.

Theoretical positions have 'real world' implications for practice, and pluralistic therapy perhaps arose out of a felt need to change therapy's theoretical foundations so that it might be provided differently, especially in a UK context. Although there is a lot of exchange between the USA and the UK amongst theoreticians, practitioners, and researchers, there are significant contextual differences, so pluralistic therapy might be seen as a geographically localised response whose importance is thus far, primarily or even exclusively, located in the UK. The agenda, fairly openly, is to change policies via practices that can be researched, using, on the whole, favoured methodologies. The end goal could be construed as ensuring more substantial influence on politically powerful providers such as NICE and the NHS, which have, up to now, in their responses to research and practice, encouraged the shutting down rather than opening up of options for therapists, clients, and researchers. However, as stated at the beginning of this chapter, these local trends I have detailed here have parallels in therapy provision throughout the Anglosphere. These details can be read like a case study by stakeholders who see in the particulars of the UK how similar processes are taking place in their own particular therapeutic and political systems.

'Pluralistic therapy' as conceptualised by Cooper and McLeod and in the increasingly numerous books and papers sparked by them is, in my view, not as important as understanding pluralism *in* therapy, *for* therapy, *in* therapists and *for* therapists. It is over fifteen years since they first formulated the idea of pluralistic therapy. Now is the time to deepen our understanding of pluralism (philosophically and politically). This can then form a basis for understanding what pluralistic practitioners as individuals or as members of groups can do to evolve the conceptualisation of a pluralistic dimension for therapy as not just a researchable approach but a philosophical and political basis for action both within and outside therapy. A pluralistic position allows for essential critiques of the current politics of therapy. These critiques need to challenge the domination of monistic cultures, which have real-world effects in limiting opportunities not just for therapists but also for the people they serve. At a minimum, those sympathetic to pluralism need to make the case that therapy is pluralistic by nature and that its pluralistic nature (i.e. the plurality of therapies) is not a weakness but a strength. Then, working outwards from the micropolitics of therapy into the macropolitics of the world, they need to challenge monistic cultures (micro and macro), which do so much to limit possibilities and potentials in a multitude of ways. Some of these latter themes will be explored further throughout the rest of the book. The philosophical and political meanings and implications of pluralism, in particular, will be explored in the following two chapters.

Chapter 3

Pluralism and Philosophy

The Meanings of Pluralism

Pluralism has a wide range of meanings and uses. In general, pluralistic paradigms advocate and encourage the acceptance of multiplicity and disagreement – 'any substantial question admits of a variety of plausible but mutually conflicting responses' (Rescher, 1993, p. 79) – and, within multiplicities, the acceptance of differing perceptions about phenomena whatever those phenomena might be. This generalised idea has been theorised and applied to particular fields such as culture, methodology, politics, religion, and philosophy. This leads to several different types of pluralism: ontological, moral-religious, value, and political, amongst many other descriptors used to specify varying angles on or refractions from the fundamental concept (e.g. Araujo & Osbeck, 2023).

Pluralism can be seen as dialectically opposite to monism in these various fields (e.g. Araujo & Osbeck, 2023; McLennan, 1995). In philosophy, the conflict between pluralism and monism goes back to ancient Greek philosophers such as Parmenides, who 'posited the essential, indivisible and eternal Oneness of being' as opposed to philosophers such as Empedocles and Democritus, who believed that 'the various elements and kinds in the world had substantial identities all of their own' (McClennan, 1995, p. 26). In relatively more recent Western philosophy, Leibniz opposed Spinoza's idea of an 'infinite, logically necessary Substance' existing in God and nature by proposing an 'infinite series of particulars' (p. 27) whose only commonality is that they are in relationship to each other.

At the turn of the 20th century, William James challenged Hegelian idealism with pluralism (2011/1908). Bertrand Russell (e.g. Russell, 1959) and James Ward (1911) also supported pluralistic positions, the latter proposing a kind of pluralism within a unifying frame, what might be termed a 'moderate' pluralism (e.g. McLennan, 1995). These philosophical inquiries into issues engendered by conceptualising monism and pluralism inform the more specialised debates about pluralism as it crosses over into other fields (McLennan, 1995).

McLennan describes pluralism as existing on three levels: 1) as a 'political science tradition of "empirical democratic theory"'(to be explored further in the next chapter); 2) as a 'more general intellectual orientation'; and 3) as a 'temperament,

DOI: 10.4324/9781003468332-3

a ... psycho-personal frame of mind' (p. 1). He suggests that pluralism is more eas-ily understood as a '"modal" concept', a way of seeing rather than a 'substantive "end-point" doctrine' to believe in (p. ix). In other words, it is a philosophy that can be applied as a way of thinking about many different theories and practices rather than necessarily encapsulating a theory and practice of its own. McLennan states that the common meaning of pluralism 'indicates our acknowledgment of multiplicity and difference across and within particular social fields and discourses' (1995). Within social science and politics, the term was formerly most associated with empirical democratic theory, which was current from the 1950s to the early 1970s (McLennan, 1995). However, since then, the word and its associated ideas have spread further into social science, politics, and other subject areas.

McLennan points out that in order to be able to comprehend potential mean-ings of pluralism we need to understand its 'conceptual opposite or "boundary condition"'(p. x). He suggests this opposite is a 'sense of unity and integration' (p. x). This point reflects an important difference between 'integrative' approaches to therapy and 'pluralistic' ones.

Another point McLennan makes, which similarly resonates with the conceptu-alisation and practice of pluralism in the 'social' field and 'discourses' of therapy, is that 'the assertion of pluralism in any particular field does not in and of itself usually produce any clear *solution*' (1995; italics in original). It might be argued, for instance, that a pluralistic perspective in the field of therapy might struggle to impact the field on any pragmatic level. The insistence of a pluralistic perspective that the answer(s) to any given question might be plural rather than singular and might be dynamic rather than static does not fit prevailing paradigms in which it is 'common sense' that there should be one answer that remains true from one year to the next. For example, the question of whether CBT is more effective than person-centred therapy is often seen by commissioning bodies as needing a binary yes/no answer. Therefore, the dominant strategy for researching therapeutic effective-ness assumes that any particular approach has a consistent 'efficacy' akin to any standardised pharmaceutical medication. A pluralistic intellectual orientation and temperament do not fit well into this prevailing modus operandi.

One charge that might be made against pluralism in many fields, including therapy, is that its flexible, accepting, inclusive nature 'appeal[s] to the overly-tolerant, *pseudo*-tolerant, ostensibly humanistic, and intellectually eclectic sort of person; the sort of person who does not really have any clear opinions on anything' (McLennan, 1995, p. 2; italics in original). The pluralistic temperament/perspec-tive in the field of therapy supports the 'dodo verdict' (e.g. Cooper, 2008; Luborsky et al., 2002; Luborsky et al., 1975; Rosenzweig, 1936) in which all must have prizes, and in which there is avoidance and fear of winners and losers. This sits within a more general poststructuralist and postmodernist paradigm in which plu-ralism in particular '[enshrines] the principle of "equal but different"'(McLennan, p. 3). McLennan (writing in 1995) calls these more postmodernist, poststructuralist meanings of pluralism a 'new pluralism' while simultaneously recognising its newness is arguable (McLennan, p. 3). The accepting, inclusive nature of pluralism has most markedly been criticised for leading to an 'anything goes' conclusion (Ayer, 1984; McLennan, 1995), since it seems to advocate a 'potentially endless multiplication of valid ideas' (McLennan, p. 8).

Wilber (2000) similarly associates 'pluralistic relativism' – although it is arguable that pluralism is relativistic (see, e.g., Connolly, 2005; Lassman, 2011) – with postmodernism. He perceives it as manifesting in particular phenomena, amongst which he includes 'Rogerian counseling' and 'humanistic psychology' (p. 50). In terms of the meanings of pluralism, it is important to emphasise how entwined it is with the meanings of postmodernism. Wilber characterises postmodernism as an '*attempt to be inclusive*' (p. 50 and italics in original). In this sense, Wilber associates postmodernism with '"diversity" (or "multiculturalism" or "pluralism")' (p. 159). His view is similar to McLennan's, who tentatively suggests that '[p]ostmodernism ... can be redescribed perhaps as the generalized affirmation of pluralism and heterogeneity' (McLennan, 1995, p. 21). Wilber, on the whole, is supportive of pluralism while criticising its potential to '[level] ... qualitative distinctions' (Wilber, 2000, p. 160). Overall, however, Wilber supports a constructivist, contextualist interpretation of reality, asserting that an integral-aperspectivist position must follow. By 'integral-aperspectivist', a term he attributes to Jean Gebser, he means 'cognition must ... unduly privilege no single perspective' (2000, p. 163). The relation of this view to how pluralism comes to be understood in the field of therapy is a close one.

Overall, pluralism refers 'to a host of interrelated issues: ontological, epistemological, methodological, ethical' (Stam, 2023, p. xi), and 'there are varieties of pluralisms and these stretch back several centuries' (p. xi). Subsequently, what we understand pluralism to mean or imply for therapy depends on the philosophical bases we embrace in our own construction of it. This will vary according to whether one prefers William James, Emmanuel Levinas, or others who have espoused different views of what pluralism might or should mean. For instance, practitioners identifying as 'pluralistic' who are more familiar with and endeared to Levinas might be more concerned with valuing the Other as a relational ethic than with valuing pluralities as such.

In a pluralistic spirit, we do not have to narrow down the meaning of pluralism to one particular field or -ology. Pluralism in relation to therapy can have meanings and implications for how we think about the plurality of approaches, the plurality of research methodologies, the plurality of providers, and the plurality of different kinds of and titles for 'mental health' practitioners and for a host of issues in which plurality can be seen as a fundamental issue or problem for the field (see Araujo & Osbeck, 2023).

William James's *A Pluralistic Universe* (1909)

William James (2011/1908) was the first author in the field of psychology to make the case for a 'pluralistic universe'. In *A Pluralistic Universe* (*APU*), based on a series of lectures he delivered in Oxford, James does not distinguish between 'humanism' and 'pluralism' (p. 3), and the main thrust of the book's argument is to argue for empiricism as opposed to idealism and rationalism. Humanism and pluralism are in direct relation because in the same way that humanism, as James interprets it, emphasises the centrality of experience over ideas, so does pluralism. The multitudinous nature of human experience does not mean that this 'pluralism' needs to be integrated into – or sourced from – one idea, such as 'God'. This leads to a stance in which the necessity for one idealistic Truth, or even 'truths', is secondary to knowledge that is gained empirically (the relation between empiricism and pluralism is acknowledged and discussed by James). Pragmatism sits comfortably with this pluralistic view, as it prioritises the utility of empirical knowledge over adhering coherently to a singular philosophy.

This pioneering work, while it might be seen as unrelated to how pluralism eventually comes to be discussed in the context of therapy, does set the markers for some current debates. For instance, on one level, it might be perceived that trials of one therapeutic approach versus another have an unproblematic basis. However, with James's work in mind, we can understand that 'ideas' about therapy are what drives much research. The unproblematic perception of aggregated, apparently unitary approaches based on ideas leads to research that, in a philosophical sense, privileges nomothetic 'top-down thinking' as opposed to an idiographic 'bottom-up' approach rooted in empirical realities. A parallel to this dichotomy in contemporary therapy research is between 'evidence-based practice' (e.g. Spring, 2007) (where, arguably, 'ideas' are pitted against each other in advance of any researched sessions taking place) versus 'practice-based evidence', in which therapeutic sessions are evaluated by instruments such as Clinical Outcomes in Routine Evaluation (CORE) forms before determining which ideas might or might not have informed those particular therapeutic sessions (e.g. Shepherd et al., 2007).

The philosophical debate at the heart of *APU* is between empiricism/pluralism, which James characterises as the 'habit of explaining wholes by parts' (p. 7), versus rationalism/monism, which James characterises as the 'habit of explaining parts by wholes' (p. 8). Again, the relevance of this text to contemporary issues in therapeutic research is similarly apparent: 'whole' approaches are evaluated as worthy or not worthy and then directed at the 'parts', namely therapists and clients in practice, for instance, with manualised treatments, whereas therapists and clients in practice as 'parts', I would suggest, are not as influential in directing how 'whole' therapies might be delivered. There has been a significant amount of 'process' research (e.g. Rhodes & Smith, 2010; Theriault & Gazzola, 2008; 2006), some of it coming from research about pluralistic therapy itself (e.g. Watson et al., 2012). However, despite the amount and quality of process research, it still does not impact decisions about policy and provision as much as the more influential symptom-driven approach of RCTs.

The tendency towards wanting definitive and timeless answers as to whether therapy A is better than therapy B also reflects an idealistic, rationalistic and monistic basis, which James challenges in this text: 'The commonest vice of the human mind is its disposition to see everything as yes or no, as black or white, its incapacity for discrimination of intermediate shades' (p. 26).

In sum, *APU* is important not just for how pluralism, in more recent times, becomes applied to the theory and practice of therapy and ideas about how therapy might conceptualise itself for future practice but also for how therapy is researched and assumptions about the validity of that research.

Isaiah Berlin (1909–1997) and Value Pluralism

Isaiah Berlin is famous for his essay 'Two Concepts of Liberty', written in 1958. In this crucial text for explorations and understandings about political freedom, he makes a 'distinction between positive and negative liberty' (Cherniss & Hardy, 2023), where negative liberty is freedom from negative things such as coercion and positive liberty is freedom towards, for example, doing as one pleases.

Generally, Berlin is concerned with 'systems of value' – what we value, the beliefs we hold, and the choices we make in living out those values and beliefs. These systems are pluralistic, just as values themselves are pluralistic, and often, to uphold one value, another value must be sacrificed. For instance, to uphold the value of liberty, the value of order or equality must sometimes be lost.

Like James, Berlin also defined pluralism as the opposite of monism. From Berlin's pluralistic perspective, there can be multiple answers to questions, multiple methods and methodologies for discovering answers *if* those answers exist, and these answers to questions do not necessarily make sense in relation to each other (i.e. there is not necessarily some overriding coherent whole to which they belong). The universe is not necessarily either harmonious or coherent (Cherniss & Hardy, 2023). This parallels a pluralistic view that dissensus, disharmony, and incoherence are not necessarily undesirable. The many arguments between proselytisers of different therapeutic approaches, which to some signify a major problem for the development of therapy, are for pluralists inevitable and potentially valuable (e.g. Rescher, 1993).

Emmanuel Levinas

Emmanuel Levinas is a central figure for many 'pluralistic therapy' practitioners in the UK. Since Cooper and McLeod (2011) first comprehensively articulated the pluralistic therapy framework, Levinas seems to have been the figure who has most influenced the philosophical spirit behind pluralistic therapy as Cooper envisions it. In 2020, in response to philosophical challenges by Ong et al. (2020), Cooper argued that the 'fundamental grounds' for his version of pluralistic therapy:

> … lie in an ethics of care. This is particularly informed by the work of the French philosopher Emmanuel Levinas. For Levinas, the fundamental philosophical question is not "What is truth?" or "What is existence?" but how can we relate to each other in caring and respectful ways: open and welcoming to the otherness of the Other.
>
> (Cooper, 2020)

In more recent years, Cooper has turned his focus towards issues around social justice, most extensively in *Psychology at the Heart of Social Change* (2023) and practically with the formation of a 'Therapy and Social Change' (TaSC) networking group. Levinas's philosophy of valuing the other is central to this intensification of a political drive, which Cooper identifies as a pluralistic value and is central to his vision of pluralistic therapy. This takes place within a context in which therapy and therapists are generally becoming more overtly political concerning the world outside the therapy room and taking on issues such as classism, racism, colonialism, and discrimination of various kinds both within and outside the therapy world, sometimes conceptualised as a politics concerned with 'intersectionality' based on personal oppressions, privileges, and identities (e.g., see Turner, 2021).

It is worth noting that the emphasis on this particular form of pluralism goes away from a more Jamesian version of pluralism, where ontology and epistemology are central concerns. In terms of therapy, who we *are*, the nature of being human (ontology), is central to therapeutic processes and goals, whether that is explicit or implicit: the more we understand who we are, the more the various therapies and therapists can claim to have clarity, coherence, and purposeful intentions – similarly, attempting to differentiate value and understand different therapies, whether by standard research methods and methodologies or via the direct phenomenological experiences of clients and therapists, is also of central concern (epistemology). In sum, a Levinasian pluralism might be said to encapsulate a meaning of pluralism that is more of a 'cause' than the more metaphysical meanings in a Jamesian pluralism (Araujo & Osbeck, 2023).

While I am sympathetic towards the political and ethical dimensions of pluralism, which are being increasingly espoused as central to Cooper and McLeod's pluralistic therapy, in many ways, it seems to me that James has more to offer (Araujo & Osbeck, 2023) because he includes within his purview of pluralism issues around ontology, epistemology, and even moral-religious pluralism. It might also be said that if the main thrust of Cooper's pluralistic therapy is a pluralism 'based on a specific value: a valuing of others and how they see the world' (Cooper, 2020), then in some ways he is only really advocating a new version of person-centred therapy (and, for example, its concept of 'unconditional positive regard'), and this tendency forms at least part of the critiques coming from person-centred adherents such as Ong et al. (2020).

Postmodernism

Various therapy approaches have been challenged by postmodernist critics, who argue against these approaches' uncritical assumptions regarding their own 'truths' and unproblematic 'modern' beliefs in a theory–practice axis (e.g. House, 2003; Parker, 1999a; 1999b; Polkinghorne, 1992). The postmodern condition is described by Polkinghorne (1992) as being one of 'foundationlessness' and 'fragmentariness'. From this point of view, the attempt to make a 'modern' sense of things, including therapy, goes against a postmodern sensibility. Jung himself said that '[t]herapy is different in every case ...psychotherapy and analysis are as varied as are human individuals' (Jung, 1963, p. 131, in Szasz, 1988, p. 175). However, modern attempts to combine the fragments of therapy into practices with theoretical foundations continue unabated, whether in the development or creation of particular schools or in attempts to theorise integrative models.

Pluralism goes against the tendency to want to make unified wholes, and so the attempt to codify a pluralistic therapy, as Cooper and McLeod have, does not sit well with some critics such as Loewenthal (2016; 2012; 2011) and House (2011) amongst others.

The importance of postmodernism in relation to pluralism and pluralistic therapy will be more thoroughly explored in Chapter 10.

Andrew Samuels

Andrew Samuels views pluralism as an 'attitude to conflict which tries to reconcile differences without imposing a false resolution on them or losing sight of the value of each position' (Samuels, 2011/1997, p. 223). His arguments might pithily be expressed by William Blake's saying that 'Without Contraries is no progression' (Blake, 1957/1790–1793, p. 149, capitalisation in original), and these contraries can remain opposed without yielding to a false unity. Similarly to McLennan (1995), he also views pluralism as a mode, process, or a 'tool or instrument' rather than a 'desirable state or goal' (Samuels, 2011/1997, p. 229). For Samuels, pluralism is not an ideal end-point for the profession but is a way of understanding and using the reality of differences for the benefit of everyone.

Mick Cooper and John McLeod

Cooper and McLeod (2007) initially situated the philosophical basis for pluralism in the work of Rescher (1993) and aligned it with postmodernism. Like McLennan (1995) and Wilber (2000), they emphasise the centrality of being inclusive in postmodern/pluralistic thinking and view this as an 'ethical and political commitment' (Cooper & McLeod, 2007, p. 136), not just at a philosophical level but also within the therapy profession towards other practitioners and clients. Cooper and McLeod further associate this understanding of pluralism 'as a form of humanistic-existential ethic' (p. 136). This explicit humanistic–existential leaning hints at a potentially problematic bias for practitioners not so broadly humanistic–existential in orientation. Similarly, those more sympathetic to the assertion that the 'principles underlying [humanistic–existential] approaches are of universal relevance to the practice of psychotherapy' (Cooper, 2007, p. 11) might find themselves more aligned with Cooper and McLeod's pluralistic ideas. The explicit humanistic–existential underpinning might also be seen as a more political move to re-brand humanistic therapies to make them more acceptable to more powerful therapy providers.

The humanistic–existential philosophical basis for their pluralistic approach might alienate practitioners who do not come from that philosophical position. Cooper and McLeod (2011) anticipate that resistance and attempt to make their humanistic position inclusive of all practitioners by framing it as a general 'ethic' rather than any specific therapeutic practice – one that might apply to any kind of therapy, including CBT. They argue that collaboration is what makes any therapy humanistic, so that even person-centred therapy, if it is delivered without client involvement, could be non-humanistic. This is a valiant attempt to bridge divides; nevertheless, it does come across as trying to claim humanistic values as more universally accepted than is perhaps the case. It might also be seen as wishful thinking that their values can be trans-theoretical when perhaps that potential is problematic and limited.

House is sceptical that Cooper and McLeod's pluralistic approach, despite allying itself with postmodernism, engages with postmodern thinking and accuses them of being more 'modern' in their 'privileging of "goals", "skills", [and] "methods"'(House, 2011). Adam Scott, similarly, states that it is 'the philosophy behind pluralism … rather than the structure of goals, tasks and methods' which grounds him (Scott & Hanley, 2012, p. 36). Scott understands the view of some therapists that pluralism makes more sense as a philosophical basis for practice rather than a prescribed way to practise (p. 39).

The pragmatic issue at stake here is that it is extremely difficult to 'test' the philosophical positions of therapists if no framework, structure, or protocols are identified as being 'pluralistic therapy'. The implications of understanding pluralism as a dimension of therapy rather than any specific practice(s) do not sit easily in the contemporary world of 'evidence-based' therapies and audit cultures.

Pluralism, Multiculturalism, and 'Cultural Pluralism'

Pluralism, as a word, is often associated with multiculturalism. Indeed, Wilber (2000), as stated earlier in this chapter, sees pluralism as synonymous with a positive vision of diversity and multiculturalism. There are, however, distinct differences between understandings of multiculturalism and 'cultural pluralism' in the literature (see Drew, 2023). Both cultural pluralism and multiculturalism envision societies 'in which multiple cultures coexist peacefully', but a 'culturally plural society has one dominant culture', whereas a 'multicultural society has no dominant culture' (Drew, 2023).

The USA is a good example of a 'culturally pluralist' society as it has myriad different cultural groups who do not necessarily assimilate their culture into the dominant culture. If a multicultural society is seen as a society in which there is 'no one dominant cultural group and widespread cultural variation' (Drew, 2023), then the USA is not currently an example, although it does have an increasing percentage of 'majority minority' cities (Drew, 2023).

When considering cultural pluralism and multiculturalism, we must also consider important differences between integration and assimilation. In integration,

wholes are not lost: in other words, one culture can exist alongside another without losing its identity. In assimilation, however, two cultures 'become similar'
(Drew, 2023). In time, they become indistinguishable, and their own identities
become lost.

Early debates about multiculturalism/cultural pluralism originated in the USA,
where, in response to the impact of mass immigration on American culture, it
was debated whether the USA was a 'melting pot' (assimilation) or a 'salad bowl'
(integration).

There are interesting metaphorical similarities between these subtly different
conceptualisations of differences applied to cultures, which can also be applied
to thinking about the plurality of therapies. For instance, it might be argued that
health providers often try to create a culturally plural (at best) rather than a multicultural provision of therapies and therapists. There is a desire for a dominant
therapeutic approach (currently CBT) and a dominant majority culture (currently a
more 'psychological' emphasis on therapy). The more psychological emphasis on
therapy devalues more 'philosophical' and 'relational' types of therapy, preferring
to privilege alleged psychological 'experts' with 'evidence-based' manuals and
protocols. Similarly, the concept of integration in thinking about cultures applied
to therapies reflects pluralistic ideals. However, the notion of a 'common factors'
therapy reaching its logical conclusions might suggest more of a 'melting pot'/
assimilation approach to the theory and practice of therapy. These arguments will
be revisited in later chapters.

In more recent years, Dwight Turner has contributed a great deal to the literature
in the areas of multiculturalism/cultural pluralism, both in terms of how these issues show up in the therapy world at different levels and also theorising at more
general philosophical and political levels about how issues of race and 'othering'
more generally affect societies as a whole (see, e.g., Turner, 2024). He recognises
that the 'Subject's idea of the Other has been a core component of philosophy for
hundreds of years' (2024, p. 94). He criticises Cartesian dualism and celebrates
philosophies which challenge it, identifying Spinoza as one of the first to do so.
Both Buber and Levinas also influence Turner. However, he feels they fall short
because they still seem to assume 'identity being … a singular construct' (2024,
p. 95). Turner asserts, 'our intersecting identities are multiple, numerous and un-
countable' (p. 95). Here, we see another facet of pluralism, in its broadest sense,
when pluralism is referring to the idea of the 'plural self' (Rowan & Cooper, 1998).
However, Turner, as far as I am aware, does not identify as a 'pluralistic' therapist
per se. Turner's philosophical speculations around intersectionality (Turner, 2021)
hold interesting parallels to pluralistic philosophy. Turner suggests that the complexities of human beings do not lend themselves to simplistic dualities of 'subject
and object, supremacy inferiority' (Turner, 2024, p. 96). He calls for thinking about
people, especially their identities, beyond dualistic notions and into the 'plural'
(p. 97). Following on from the idea of a plural self comes the conceptualisation
of multiple 'parts' in the psyche (an idea that goes back to the very beginnings of
therapy but which has become popularised most recently with the 'internal family

systems' theory). Turner suggests it is the most wounded intersectional identities or parts that, as it were, end in therapy.

Ultimately, Turner uses these philosophical foundations to make strong political arguments against supremacy, not just in terms of race but in a host of intersections. In the next chapter, there is more to say about his ideas in relation to pluralism from a political perspective, in which recent articulations about social justice and intersectionality – concepts connected to multiculturalism but not the same – will be explored amongst other issues concerning more political meanings of pluralism.

Chapter 4

Pluralism and Politics

This chapter explores pluralism as it is conceptualised politically in a general sense, as well as particular meanings and associations with social justice and intersectionality. Once the fundamentals of these concepts have been sufficiently discussed, the chapter will explore some implications of pluralism for the micropolitical world of therapy from a macropolitical perspective.

Pluralism: Political Conceptualisations

Pluralism as a political idea has held sway most strongly in the USA and the UK. In the USA, it mainly refers to a political system in which there is an assumption that 'all political parties have a right to exist' and that there will be a 'peaceful rotation of power' (Muasher, 2014). It also refers to a plurality of power centres. These power centres might be geographical, from within a central legislature such as Congress in Washington, alongside regional power centres such as state legislatures. Similarly, power is also held by various judicial systems, which are theoretically independent of the government.

Additionally, within the pluralistic ideal, the ambition that people form interest groups of various kinds, most obviously unions but also lobby and pressure groups, adds to the plurality of ways people can seek and express power over their lives. In the UK, pluralism – as a political concept – holds similar meanings but with more of an emphasis on unions facilitating non-governmental, community-based modes of power. Pluralism in the UK is more associated with the left, particularly Labour Party figures such as Harold Laski and G.D.H. Cole (Reid, 2002).

With a political pluralistic perspective applied to therapy, we can ask questions such as 'How is power distributed in therapy systems?' from the smallest therapy dyad of therapist and client across to unions (if they exist), training and educational providers, professional associations, pressure groups, healthcare systems, third sector organisations, up to political organisations and representatives legislating for the public. If all these groups of people within the therapy world are perceived to be much the same as interest groups within the wider world, then we can see that, in terms of policy, they may well have different preferences, which lead to at least some of the debates within the profession, most significantly in terms of how the

DOI: 10.4324/9781003468332-4

profession evolves in relation to professionalisation and regulation. These themes will be explored both in this chapter and throughout the book.

In the USA, a pluralistic political system is contrasted with a political system controlled by elites (e.g. Mills, 1956). It could be argued that this pluralism versus elitism dynamic is intensely present in the professionalisation of therapy. Regular, persistent, and ever-changing methods of institutionalising the perceived superiority/inferiority of different types of therapists manifest alongside a simultaneous fight-back from at least some therapists resisting this process. This drive for superiority is seen by Turner (2024) as foundational to the phenomenon of supremacy in terms of race, class, gender, and other intersections. I would suggest this drive for superiority is also found in the diversity of therapists (as defined by various intersections) and their expressed, perhaps heartfelt and embodied allegiances to theoretical approaches.

William Connolly and the 'New Pluralism'

William Connolly (2005), in his critical engagements with pluralism as a political concept, has created what some call a 'new pluralism' (Campbell & Schoolman, 2008). This new pluralism contrasts with a more conventional 'old pluralism' as it has been more commonly understood in political science and sociology since the Second World War. Connolly incorporates ideas from poststructuralism, postmodernism, critical theory, and feminism to update and critique conventional interpretations of pluralistic politics, especially within the context of the USA (Schoolman & Campbell, 2008a). Connolly's new pluralism 'aims to ... [think] critically about existing political constellations and the multiple ways in which they can be reconfigured' (p. 1).

He identifies the 'bias of pluralism' (Connolly, 1969). This bias manifests as the embedded notion amongst many pluralistic theorists that pluralism is reflective of contemporary American politics and society – and proof of its democratic foundations – when, in fact, it is maybe better thought of as an ideal which has not been attained and as something which democratic political processes will be forever working towards.

Connolly roots pluralistic ideals in Tocqueville, who wrote about American democracy in the early 19th century (Schoolman & Campbell, 2008a). Comparing the pluralistic ideals of Tocqueville to the realities of modern democratic societies reveals various shortcomings: 1) citizens from all classes and ranks are not participating in politics, 2) voluntary associations which Tocqueville viewed as 'vehicles for political education, for safeguarding rights and for aggregating and articulating political demands' are actually 'compromised by modern, large-scale organizations whose structural dynamics favor oligarchical interests over those of an organization's membership' (2008a, p. 3), 3) there are few who have the time and ability to be active in such associations, and 4) the media does not represent a plurality of views but instead reflects similar views 'by economic elites' (2008a). These factors demonstrate that modern democracies fall short of a pluralistic ideal as envisioned by Tocqueville and others. The critiques of those assuming an actual pluralistic reality rather than an ideal are summed up by Connolly as reflecting a 'critical temper' typically found on the left and especially in the social sciences (2008a). These left-leaning social scientists contrast markedly with those who 'assume the legitimacy of the dominant values' (2008a, p. 6). Pluralism in politics, therefore, becomes an ideal to aim for and a political philosophy that can be used to critique the successes and failings of incomplete pluralising processes, not just in their 'being' but also in their 'becoming' (Schoolman & Campbell, 2008b).

One concept central to Connolly's concerns is what he phrases as the 'power of the evangelical-capitalist resonance machine'. What he means by this is that he does not believe that evangelical Christians have taken over the Republican Party or, conversely, that the Republican Party is manipulating evangelical Christians for its own gain but rather that both groups resonate with each other and are so folded into each other that there is no simple reciprocity or simple unified ideology. Rather, it is more like a Jungian complex, both metaphorically and in the sense that these resonances between different groups are often unconscious, unarticulated, and allied to feelings along with personal and collective narratives. The evangelical–capitalist resonance machine is just one example of the different types of combinations that exist in the world (Schoolman & Campbell, 2008b).

Aligning with Connolly's analysis of an evangelical–capitalist resonance machine is his emphasis that ordinary political concepts 'such as power, interests, legitimacy, freedom, democracy – and politics itself – express deeper onto-religious differences' (2008b, p. 306). This perception can easily be applied to the world of therapy, not only in the multitude of approaches which attract evangelised adherents but, importantly, in the more fundamental divide between those who have an onto-religious sensibility towards therapy as an 'art' versus those who either see therapy as already having attained or want it to attain someday the status of being a 'science'. This latter split in the profession is as polarised as any left/right differences in the more general political sphere, although less well articulated and discussed. These firmly held beliefs, although sometimes established upon or supported by empirical evidence, more often than not actually appeal to personal preferences regarding metaphorical models of the psyche and interpersonal relationships. Whether therapists prefer to talk about the 'ego' rather than the 'Adult', the 'unconscious' rather than 'outside awareness' and so forth, is mostly a matter of taste rather than anything truly 'evidence-based'. The profoundly important differences between the push for therapy to be classified and practised as a science versus the understanding of therapy as more of an art/craft rooted in uncertainty and creativity will be discussed throughout this book with the more specific concerns therapists have about their identities, especially as defined by adherence to approaches, explored in the next chapter.

Of course, nothing stands still, and Connolly brings to bear on pluralism the ever-increasing speed of change over time. This means that any assumed centre of power is continually challenged by peripheral groups who either exist already or are coming into being. These contestations for power are also easily observed in the field of therapy. From this standpoint, it can be helpful to differentiate pluralism as it might now exist with a pluralising process that is forever evolving. Connolly identifies 'emerging constituencies' who 'allow a new identity, right, good or faith to cross the threshold of legitimacy' (2008b, p. 307). The challenges of these constituencies – in the therapy world – to mainstream definitions, constructions, and assumptions about therapy become more intense and frequent. The wish to define and set standards for therapy as well as having benign intentions might also be seen as a conservative, reactionary defence by the 'old guard'; an attempt to institutionalise therapy before new entrants have the chance to tear down any favoured existing structures.

Connolly also uses the postmodern concepts of 'micropolitics' as opposed to the 'macropolitics' of governments and political assemblies. How both philosophical and political interpretations of pluralism can be applied to the micropolitical world of therapy is of central concern, explicitly or implicitly, throughout this book.

Pluralism as a political concept reflects my position towards pluralism in therapy: that is, for me, pluralism is not so important as a framework under which to bring together a collection of techniques and/or approaches, such as Cooper and McLeod's 'pluralistic therapy' (e.g. Cooper & McLeod, 2011), but is better understood as a dimension of therapy which can act as a basis for understanding therapy's potentials from a philosophical and political viewpoint, especially in terms of how these understandings might manifest themselves in the concrete world.

Pluralism, Social Justice, and Intersectionality

Social Justice

Bell (2016) defines social justice as the 'full and equal participation of people from all social identity groups in a society'. Furthermore, Bell states that the pursuit of this ideal goal 'should also be democratic and participatory, respectful of human diversity and group differences, and inclusive and affirming of human agency and capacity for working collaboratively with others to create change' (Bell, 2016, p. 3). The parallels with therapy, especially an explicitly pluralistic therapy, are apparent as pluralistic therapy (Cooper & McLeod, 2011) emphasises that collaboration between clients and therapists forms part of the core of any kind of therapy considering itself to be pluralistic. The foundational idea is that because clients are not homogeneous, then it is unlikely that the same approach (named or otherwise) will be effective with all. This leads to offering an array of therapeutic options as the best logical outcome of the premise. However, this conclusion is profoundly different to those of therapy providers, who often aim to minimise options or have no options at all other than, for example, CBT. It is highly arguable that this embedded attitude respects 'human diversity' and 'group differences'. Conversely, the overarching goal of social justice to 'create change' at the macro scale is, of course, reflected at the micro scale in therapy. Unsurprisingly, Charura and Winter (2023) acknowledge that Cooper and McLeod's pluralistic therapy aligns well with principles of social justice. Gabriel (2023) suggests that other features of pluralistic therapy, namely case formulation, working with client preferences, and metacommunication, also fit a social justice agenda in therapy.

Intersectionality

Intersectionality is described by Patricia Hill Collins and Sirma Bilge (2020) as:

> investigat[ing] how intersecting power relations influence social relations across diverse societies as well as individual experiences in everyday life. As an analytical tool, intersectionality views categories of race, class, gender, sexuality, nation, ability, ethnicity and age – among others – as interrelated and mutually shaping one another. Intersectionality is a way of understanding and explaining complexity in the world, in people and human experiences.
>
> (p. 2 cited in Lago, 2023, p. 29)

As Lago (2023) suggests, this is different to the meanings and intentions of multiculturalism. Intersectionality is explicitly concerned with 'inequalities embedded within society' (p. 29), usually in terms of perceiving privilege and oppression in the various categories.

Turner (2024), following on from Collins (2019), emphasises three major intersections of privilege and oppression, namely capitalism, patriarchy, and white supremacy. These three can be viewed independently, but Turner suggests it is more helpful to view them all as profoundly interconnected and relevant to everyone, whether privileged or oppressed, in any given category.

Turner further suggests that the 'internalised supremacist is a massive aspect of who we all are' because '[a]s part of our superego, it helps us to form our identity, it builds us up and it creates images, examples of who we believe we happen to be in relation to others' (Turner, 2024, p. 7). He conceptualises it in relation to a fear-driven 'Superiority Drive' (p. 94).

This superiority drive – which is directly linked to the supremacies of capitalism, patriarchy, and white supremacy – can also be seen at play in all kinds of varying contexts. Turner conceptualises that around the perceived 'superior' position, such as a patriarch, there are concentric circles starting with 'acolytes', moving to 'outliers' and only in the outer ring does the truly 'other' exist. The centre illustrates the 'central ideology, person, or institution', and the '[a]colytes are those people who will sit around that central position and maintain their superiority' (2024, p. 90). They do so by projecting onto the central 'superior' ideas of 'goodness … [m]orality and … rightness' (p. 90). The centre also encourages the acolytes to remain close by, as they seem to offer safety. Thus, the acolytes 'give up their own authenticity and centrality and become part of a co-opted centre' (p. 90). Turner discusses these ideas in relation to major issues around race, class, and various oppressions. However, the similarities with therapy 'schools'/approaches and the seeming safety offered to practitioners and the public by membership bodies and so forth are striking. The term 'acolyte' also echoes Connolly's perception of onto-religious sensibilities informing political allegiances, which similarly seem to be echoed in therapists' allegiances to their own centres. Arguably, similar effects of giving up one's authenticity to be allowed into the fold and not seen as 'other' run deep within the therapy field.

Implications for Therapy

The Art/Science Divide, the Medical Model, and the Politics of Research

As stated in a previous section, there is an intense, political, and fundamental di-vide within the therapy professions. This divide is between those who see therapy as more of an art/craft rooted in uncertainty and creativity versus those who either think therapy has already attained and deserves the status of being a science (and/or medical procedure) or needs to do all it can to get there. The latter tend to be more supportive of the medical model and its application to therapy in terms of how it is provided – the medical model being the assumption that therapy is a medical 'treatment' and, as such, needs to be based on diagnosis–treatment–cure. This is what Rowan (2005b) describes as an 'instrumental' attitude towards therapy as opposed to a 'relational' one.

Many practitioners are uncomfortable with the medical model's increasingly hegemonic dominance over the conceptualisation and practice of therapy. From a pluralistic perspective, there can be a 'both/and' solution to these opinionated dif-ferences. For instance, in terms of collaboration, central to the practice of pluralis-tic therapy, it is not up to the therapist to impose a medical or non-medical view on or about the client. If a client wants to understand their depression as based in biol-ogy, no matter what the practitioner thinks of that view, if they are flexible, they can allow the client, in person-centred terms, to inhabit their own frame of reference, even if they have concerns or doubts about that frame of reference. Simultaneously, it would be beholden on more medically-minded practitioners not to insist on cli-ents (or 'patients') conforming to their medicalised views of client problems unless the person actually wants to be 'treated' in that way. Ultimately, deep philosophi-cal positions are being held here that are highly dependent on practitioners' views about the nature of bodies and minds. It might be that some clients need more of an art/relational versus a science/instrumental approach. Only with a pluralistic perspective will clients be able to access the therapy they want and prefer.

The art/science divide in the therapy professions is also felt in practitioners' relationship to research. This is sometimes in relation to research in general, which often seems irrelevant to therapists' actual practice, and sometimes this is in rela-tion to perceived injustices such as specific methodologies, usually quantitative, being privileged above qualitative research, no matter how thorough, rigorous, and comprehensive that qualitative research might be.

Attempts were made and continue to be made to bridge the practitioner/ researcher divide in the therapy profession by encouraging the idea of 'practitioner research' (e.g. McLeod, 1999). However, whether more practitioner researchers have influenced significant change in how providers evaluate therapy is a moot point. The hope that practice-based evidence (PBE) (e.g. Lees & Freshwater, 2008) might be valued as much as evidence-based practice (EBP) still seems some way off being realised (e.g. Hanley & Winter, 2016), with RCTs especially, at the top of the hierarchy of credibility with bodies such as NICE. This reflects the current 'politics of research' (Parker, 2015).

Cooper and McLeod's (2007) original paper, promoting a pluralistic framework, is subtitled 'Implications for Research', which points to their ideas about and for therapy to be conceptualised in ways that make being researchable its central concern. This may seem prima facie unproblematic. However, it is also indicative of a profession subservient to research-driven and political agendas – most implicitly the need for approaches, including Cooper and McLeod's newly articulated framework – to prove themselves as efficacious and effective to assume or retain professionally powerful and respectable status.

The disconnect between the practice of research and practitioners' empirical understanding is widening. This has enormous political implications in terms of the power dynamics within the profession.

Counselling, Psychotherapy, and Different Approaches

It often seems to practitioners that the dice are loaded. For instance, there is very little (if any) evidence which finds any substantial differences between 'counselling' and 'psychotherapy', yet there is a persistent insistence from various stakeholders that there are differences. These beliefs lead to one of the many therapy 'wars' (to be explored further in Chapter 8).

From the beginning of my training, when I started to meet other practitioners in a pre-professional way, and since qualification over 25 years ago, I have witnessed the manifestation of 'therapy wars' in my social and professional interactions (personal and intellectual) around titles, professionalisation, and regulation, especially in relation to approach but also in the context of political struggles. Are different approaches to therapy really that different, or are they just socially constructed to be different to stake out political/economic territories? How do therapists and their seeming allies compete for various kinds of status and power?

Different therapies often seem to have different names for the same thing and are just repackaged for political and economic purposes. In the literature, most notably in Miller, Duncan and Hubble's *Escape from Babel*, which sought to create a 'unifying language for psychotherapy practice' (Miller et al., 1997), the authors illustrate how therapeutic orientations sometimes struggle to distinguish themselves from each other yet still insist on doing so for political and economic reasons. However, the authors claim that 'words are practically all that separates the models from each other' (p. 11).

Professionalisation and Regulation

House and Totton (2011; 1997) emphasise the importance of pluralism for therapeutic practice in their book *Implausible Professions: Arguments for Pluralism and Autonomy in Psychotherapy and Counselling*, especially regarding issues of professionalisation, regulation, and other political aspects of therapy.

House (2011), in a letter to the BACP members' magazine *Therapy Today*, offers a multiplicity of critiques. However, his main criticism of Cooper and McLeod (2011) is that they do not engage with the '*politics* of the psychological therapies' (House, 2011, italics in original) and the 'audit culture' which surrounds it (House, 2011), particularly regarding issues of professionalisation and regulation. House also suggests Cooper and McLeod are 'perhaps ... reproducing ... quasi-"schoolist" political manoeuvrings' (2011).

CBT

CBT has taken a hegemonic position in the field of therapy, and Cooper and McLeod's (2011) pluralistic therapy could be seen as a valiant attempt to create an evidence base for non-CBT therapies. To many non-CBT practitioners, it seems that there is a need to compete – in terms of research – with CBT. The dominance of CBT is of significant concern for those not aligned with the approach. Cooper has said that 'to some extent' pluralistic practice is a political move against the dominance of CBT, but it is more of a 'move against the dominance and dogma of any one therapy' (Cooper, 2017). Ultimately, his position is that CBT is 'neither "the answer" or [sic] "the problem"'(2017).

Therapists owe it to their clients and the political implications of therapy to fight attempts to disempower practitioners in how they practise. The articulation of definitions of standards, ethics, and other issues must be co-created by the 'community of practice' (Wenger, 1997). Organisations such as the BACP could innovate more democratic and dialogical methods of policymaking and representation rather than acting in ways that mirror the same anxieties prone to befall other professional organisations. Pluralistic therapy has offered a framework by which practitioners might find a way to empower themselves with research and provision structures as they exist now. However, it does not challenge the assumptions of those structures in themselves.

Although some therapists are committed to political causes in the broadest sense in terms of initiating social change, social justice, and working towards equal opportunity, and perceive therapy as part of these broader processes (see, for example, the organisation Psychotherapists and Counsellors for Social Responsibility – PCSR), for the most part I wonder about the extent to which the majority of therapists are politically disengaged. Perhaps not feeling a need to unite as a movement to protect and develop their political interests is one reason they have become so easily disempowered, although the Psychotherapy and Counselling Union (PCU) points to the possibility of an emerging movement towards solidarity.

In this sense, the best way forward for pluralism in therapy is to re-vision itself as a political movement for change in the commissioning and provision of therapies. The independent/private sector is de facto pluralistic in that pluralistic/integrative/ eclectic practitioners can be easily identified and accessed, and clients are also free to choose from a vast array of therapists and therapies. So, at present, the private sector is effectively the refuge for clients and therapists who believe in pluralistic therapy as a perspective and practice. The sectors in which pressure needs to be applied are the public sector – in which all types of counselling and psychotherapy are being marginalised by other professionals and paraprofessionals – and the third sector, which can fall prey to mirroring the policies and procedures of the public sector.

Cooper and McLeod's Pluralistic Therapy

I hold contradictory biases about pluralism and therapy. On the one hand, I understand the deep and conscientious motives behind the call for pluralism. On the other, I understand more cynical views of it as a pragmatic, political move with relatively shallow ambitions of getting different therapies back into mainstream delivery.

In my view, the protocols for the practice of pluralistic therapy have evolved from disconnecting with the philosophy of pluralism and a misunderstanding of pluralism as equivalent to integration. McLennan's view is that the 'conceptual opposite' of pluralism is 'a sense of unity and integration' (McLennan, 1995, p. x), which makes the conflation of pluralistic therapy with integrative therapy problematic. Cooper, McLeod, and those connected with them still seem confused about this issue – sometimes trying to differentiate pluralistic therapy as something different to integrative therapy and sometimes quite casually stating that pluralistic therapy is an integrative therapy. The distinct philosophical positions of pluralism and integrationism could lead to very different political outcomes. For instance, an integrationist stance could ultimately lead to the validation of a generic 'therapy' informed by 'evidence-based' interventions. In contrast, a pluralistic stance would always celebrate and value having a multiplicity of approaches.

First and foremost, pluralism is a philosophy that Cooper and McLeod have applied to therapy on two levels. The first level is that of practice: while I understand the pragmatic attempts to explain and codify a 'pluralistic therapy', this runs the danger of creating yet another monistic way of practising. For instance, the literature and trainings about pluralistic practice have led to implicit 'rules'. When I attended the 'First International Conference on Pluralistic Counselling and Psychotherapy', most delegates seemed to assume that pluralistic therapy is grounded in the idea of goals, tasks and methods – a kind of 'Holy Trinity' for pluralistic therapy. This is one way of conceptualising it, but it is open to legitimate critique: the language does not sit easily with some practitioners. The second level on which pluralism is applied to pluralistic therapy is as a perspective: this usually makes more sense to practitioners. That perspective is what practitioners and researchers would be better focussed on to build a political movement supporting patient and client choice. A politicisation of pluralism/pluralistic therapy, as well as helping clients, is also vital to stem the tide of redundancies, underemployment, and unemployment of therapists, which is reaching crisis proportions and urgently needs to be addressed. For instance, the exploitation of qualified volunteers has been embedded into the public and third sectors and needs at least some reforms.

I am sympathetic towards a pluralistic perspective to inform practice and as a broader political position to hold in the therapy field. I see Cooper and McLeod's particular version of 'pluralistic therapy' as just one of several versions of different therapies which are pluralistic in nature. Pluralism might be considered the umbrella term to hold not just pluralistic therapy (named as such) but also these other therapies. For example, writers such as Wilber (e.g. 1979; 2000) also articulate pluralistic perspectives about therapy without using the label 'pluralistic therapy'. It is more beneficial to consider 'pluralism' as a dimension of therapy and therapists rather than a distinct approach. I see the concept of pluralism as most valuable for metatheoretical explorations (instead of trying to be a self-contained theory) and as a potential focal point to encourage political solidarity amongst therapists.

Chapter 5

Therapeutic Approaches and Identities

The therapy profession is riddled with problems of identity, professional status, and differentiations of roles and approaches. The publication of Cooper and McLeod's (2011) book *Pluralistic Counselling and Psychotherapy* intensified the controversy of these debates around various issues, such as whether some approaches are superior to others and whether practitioners should identify with only one approach or integrate different ones. While integrative therapy has a long history – and differences between integrative and pluralistic therapy, if any, will be discussed in a later section and throughout this book – Cooper and McLeod provided a focal point for a new 'pluralistic' agenda.

A common way of viewing the development of therapy has been to divide it into three major 'umbrella' approaches: 1) the psychoanalytic/psychodynamic, 2) the behavioural/cognitive–behavioural and 3) the humanistic/existential (e.g. Milne, 2003). Some commentators will also add: 4) the transpersonal (e.g. Rowan, 2005a). And within these broad categories sit an array of at least 500-plus therapeutic approaches that identify themselves as coherent and singular.

Some therapists casually work across approaches, but others insist on the rightness of their single approach without 'contamination' from other ideas that are perceived as inconsistent with their model. Sometimes, the motives for these positionings are deeply reflective and expressive of practitioners' values – and sometimes the motives may simply be commercial and status-driven.

Counselling, Psychotherapy, Approaches, and Identities

Holding tightly to particular approaches is inextricably linked to practitioners' sense of identity. Even the most open-minded therapist will have their favoured approaches and be prejudiced against others. For instance, some practitioners are openly antipathetic towards specific approaches such as CBT or psychodynamic therapy.

However, when looking at the conceptualisation of therapeutic approaches more critically, the actuality of how therapists practise fundamentally challenges the notion that identifying approaches as singular and forming coherent wholes

DOI: 10.4324/9781003468332-5

is unproblematic. Named therapies are not uniformly generic: the PCA has been theorised as having several tribes (e.g. Sanders, 2012); there are a host of different positions to be held in psychodynamic practice; 'humanistic' is an umbrella term for a whole variety of approaches/ideas; and CBT, apparently the best 'evidence-based therapy', has within its fold the essentially contradictory approaches of its 'second wave', which emphasises changing thoughts, feelings, and behaviours versus its 'third wave', which emphasises a more detached 'acceptance' of thoughts, feelings, and behaviours (i.e. mindfulness), which are two very different ways of viewing 'problems'.

There is also the issue of how large numbers of therapists who identify with single approaches but derive their practice from more than one approach support the contention that there is a gap between espoused theories (how therapists think they practise) and how they actually do practise (e.g. Thoma and Cecero, 2009). The difficulty in defining 'counselling' and 'psychotherapy' – and in identifying the extent to which there are any substantial differences between them – is also problematic not just in terms of clarity for therapists and clients but also in attempts to develop the regulation and professionalisation of these activities (discussed in the next section). Some practitioners accept a differentiation (e.g. McLeod, 2013, pp. 31–34) by characterising 'counselling' as pluralistic/eclectic in contrast to 'psychotherapy', characterised as more theory-driven and singular. However, 'counsellors' are just as likely to identify with particular approaches as 'psychotherapists' and usually identify with exactly the same approaches.

Fixed identities and approaches are difficult to hold on to because there are contradictions and confusions, even within a singular label like 'person-centred'. For instance, the meaning of a label can be loosely interpreted, which creates the potential for other approaches to come into a nominally single approach. This confusion problematises identities and approaches, as it is possible for practitioners to identify and theorise themselves as, for example, 'person-centred' yet practise in a way that other therapists might describe as 'integrative', 'eclectic', or 'pluralistic'.

Superiority/Inferiority

Over the years, I have been uncomfortable with practitioners whom I perceived as feeling superior to others because they have trained in particular approaches or they have assumed particular titles after training (e.g. 'psychotherapists' often feel more qualified than 'counsellors' even if the 'counsellors' have decades of experience and additional trainings). This superiority/inferiority complex parallels how Turner (2024) explicates the roots of supremacist thinking and relies on much the same psychology of feelings of belonging or not belonging to various in-groups and out-groups. It may be argued that it is inconsequential when applied to a privileged profession, but how healthy is it for practitioners to mirror these kinds of politics within their professional structures?

Professionalisation, Regulation, Approaches, and Identities

Objections to regulation include arguments that as soon as there are strict rules about how to practise based on what has come before then creativity and innovation are discouraged, and certain types of therapy would become disadvantaged if they did not conform to regulations (e.g. House & Totton, 1997). In addition, if a type of practice did not conform to the language used by regulatory bodies, it would be excluded. Hence, it could be argued that there are distinct threats to a more pluralistic perspective to therapy from regulation, particularly if it is insensitive to – or ignorant of – the varying needs and values of different approaches. Nevertheless, those in favour of regulation argue that it only seeks to protect the public and encourages innovation.

CBT

CBT can be likened to the 'elephant in the room' for the pluralistic agenda. Influential stakeholders highly favour it, and in terms of public relations, it has made remarkable achievements in influencing the media, usually uncritically, to accept it as the only evidence-based therapeutic approach for a wide array of disorders. Simultaneously, it has come under attack from therapists who do not follow the approach, perhaps with some rationality but also with emotional defensiveness (e.g. Leader, 2008). For therapists who do not follow the approach and believe in the efficacy of their own non-CBT approaches, it can seem like watching helplessly as one pupil gets all the prizes.

In audit cultures (e.g. King & Moutsou, 2010), which base their decisions about therapy provision on narrow definitions of evidence, it easily follows, from a pluralistic perspective, that a monistic hegemony comes into being such as CBT has in therapy. It is well known amongst therapy professionals that CBT has come to dominate provision in public health services. However, it is questionable, with evidence to support other approaches and interventions, as to why CBT should have such a hegemonic presence.

The assumption that some approaches are better than others inevitably leads to 'winners' and 'losers'. For the winners such as CBT – as an approach and CBT practitioners as a group – to support the principles of pluralism could threaten their current advantage in the field.

Approaches as Languages

At heart, therapy can be conceived of as an activity in which both the client and the therapist have different languages to symbolise their perspectives on reality in their interaction. This interaction can be theorised as a *symbolic interaction* (Blumer, 1986/1969). In other words, therapeutic activity can be interpreted, in theoretical terms, almost wholly via a symbolic interactionist lens. With a symbolic interactionist interpretation of therapy, we can understand therapists and clients as relational beings making sense of themselves in a relationship. This is the core of therapy, and everything else that may be said about it revolves around that central conceptualisation (e.g. Scott, 2015). From this perspective, therapeutic approaches – as much as they inform therapy sessions at all – are like languages which either help or hinder therapists and clients in their interactions.

Research, Approaches, and Identities

The emphasis on particular approaches forming a basis in research for 'evidence' is not one which is always shared by practitioners. The assumption that practitioners are most concerned with their identifying label, arguably, does not travel down to how frontline practitioners actually practise. In that sense, there is far too much concern with labels in mainstream research.

This is a common theme in the literature about therapy research, but although this is well-known and commonly discussed amongst practitioners, most researchers and commissioning bodies still insist on comparing therapeutic approaches over other variables.

The dominance of this approach-based research, when other research seems to demonstrate that it is misplaced (see Cooper, 2008), is a cause of anger for therapists and fuels debates about pluralism and therapy.

Therapists themselves do not conceptualise different approaches as that central to effectiveness, and it is no wonder that they are frustrated by the dubious basis of research that insists on attempting to compare approaches rather than the qualities of the therapists delivering those approaches.

However, such views do not easily fit into a system in which therapeutic procedures must be codified and manualised to validate particular approaches. In any case, research demonstrates that therapists (at least outside the constraints of a clinical trial) often do not practise in accordance with the principles of their identified approach (Thoma & Cecero, 2009). Additionally, the evidence gathered by clinical trials in favour of particular approaches is somewhat blighted by the phenomenon of 'researcher allegiance' (Mearns et al., 2013, p. 189).

Thus, there are a multitude of paradoxes, contradictions, and misunderstandings in how therapists identify with approaches, which problematises research based on comparing them: the notion of therapists adhering to a given approach is, at best, slippery.

Nevertheless, research that is taken seriously usually conforms to the protocol of comparing one approach against another or proving the effectiveness of an apparently consistently delivered unitary approach. This is despite the likelihood that practitioners who identify with a particular approach, especially those with more experience, will vary widely in how they practise. For the sake of a successful RCT, differences between them must be minimised or eliminated.

This illustrates a further problem in that researchers (including those nominally sympathetic to – and within – the profession) continue to push for 'technical' knowledge about practice, conforming to the demand of the medical model that not only should specific approaches be identified for specific disorders but also that specific interventions and processes should be identified for best practice within sessions, while practitioners themselves often emphasise the relational aspects of therapy above the technical. It seems the disconnect between the practice of research and practitioners' empirical understanding is widening.

Furthermore, if it is problematic for approaches to be strictly defined and/or manualised, and if, over time, practitioner experience leads to a more eclectic/ pluralistic practice, then RCTs and their strict criteria for defining approaches might be seen as only applicable to less skilled and less experienced practitioners.

Training/Education, Supervision, Approaches, and Identities

Most therapy trainings are usually rooted in one approach, even if that approach is 'integrative' or 'pluralistic'. This contrasts with the training of counselling psychologists, who must be familiar with at least two models. Training in only one approach sets up the conditions for an identity based on only one approach. Indeed, there is often an explicit or implicit assumption in therapy trainings that trainees should focus on just one approach so that their training leaves them with an unconfused and coherent view of how to practise therapy (e.g. Feltham, 2011/1997).

Most therapists identify with the approach in which they were trained. Some stay close to their original training, and it continues to significantly influence their practice. However, many therapists evolve into practising very differently from the approach of their original training. Sometimes, it is quite nuanced: it might be that practitioners still identify with the approach of their first training and, in some ways, stay close to it but in other ways go off-piste quite easily with no compunction about doing so.

The practitioner's identity/approach is usually relatively unchallenged in training. Even if the course encourages critical thinking, it will inherently believe in its own value and, therefore, implicitly encourage and inculcate its own concepts and values. Therefore, in therapy trainings, the trainees and tutors often have a cosy consensus about the 'rightness' of their particular approach.

When training, it is not surprising that often trainees will not be that confident about their practical abilities and theoretical knowledge. So, there is a kind of refuge and feeling of safety in subscribing to the approach being taught – as long as the trainee sticks to the 'rules', they will be okay, and all will be well regarding effectiveness and ethics. It is not difficult to then take that feeling of security that the approach offers and believe that it is the best approach and that other approaches do not measure up to the principles and practices of one's own. Furthermore, if other practitioners/people/providers do not like or understand the approach, there is something wrong with them rather than with the practitioner or the approach.

In addition, many trainees intensely identify with the approach they train in. In that way, it is not just a collection of techniques or a comprehensive theory with which to embark on a career but something more personal – for many, it becomes a key component of one's identity, a way of understanding the self (see the next section for more on this), world, and others and a philosophy to live by – and, in that sense, something one might not want to leave/lose or even sully with ideas and practices that come from elsewhere.

Supervision, especially group supervision (which trainees often have), is a site where practitioners are influenced by their experience of learning about different approaches, and they can be challenged about commitment or lack of commitment to their own training's approach. Group supervision can be hostile towards approaches seen as 'other' to one's own. If, for example, the supervisor holds to a specific approach at odds with the trainee's, then this can be problematic if the trainee thinks that what they are reporting is demonstrative of good work but the supervisor sees it differently not because of ability but because of theoretical differences.

However, more positively, group supervision can also be a place where the plurality of different views, experiences, and approaches can act as lenses through which to see how therapy practice can be conceptualised in many different ways. This can be a precious and valuable experience in which people contribute from a variety of models in order to understand therapeutic processes. Whether individual or group, supervision is a significant site of contestation for more or less pluralistic and puristic attitudes to therapy to be explored and developed.

The initial training in which practitioners qualify can also lead to the initial identity label of a practitioner for purely professional purposes. Technically, the therapist is only qualified in the therapy they have trained in, so most therapists will only feel comfortable using that identity label. Moreover, whether the therapist is aiming for employment or self-employment, some kind of descriptor for the therapy practised is usually required. Even if the newly qualified therapist is unsure or confused about the identification that has been bestowed upon them, it is professionally advantageous to identify with the term that has been assigned to one's training and, perhaps, ethically dubious to claim experience or knowledge of other approaches outside of that training. It is also possible that practitioners identify with a particular approach because that is the title of the qualification rather than as a deeply felt identification with the approach itself.

At later stages, additional trainings and CPD (which practising therapists are required to undertake) have a strong potential to influence a practitioner's approach. For most practitioners, over time, there is a fluidity of identity and approach in their practice, and many practitioners stray from their original training. Other influences besides supervision which impact therapists and influence their practice outside of an original training include broadly therapeutic experiences, other professional experiences, personal therapy, and literature.

However, some practitioners stay very close to the theoretical and practical bases of their original trainings, so I postulate a 'purist–pluralist continuum': some therapists are more at one end than the other, but hardly any therapists are absolutely pluralist or absolutely purist. It is also notable that the labels such as 'CBT' or 'person-centred' are themselves fluid and subject to change over time and in different contexts.

Some practitioners connect deeply, not just to the pragmatic aspects of the approaches in which they have trained, but to the philosophical foundations of those approaches. The push for more generic types of therapy, based on not just evidence-based approaches but evidence-based interventions within therapeutic sessions, threatens to undermine approaches with strong theoretical foundations for working with clients in idiosyncratic ways (such as the psychodynamic and person-centred approaches). Pluralistic therapy offers a both/and solution in which therapists can strongly identify with particular approaches if they want to, without simultaneously needing to hold a position that devalues those that are pragmatic, eclectic, or integrative.

Sense of Self, Approaches, and Identities

Sometimes, therapists have a relatively static sense of identity and approach. For some therapists, there is a connection between who they feel themselves to be and their approach. For instance, person-centred practitioners often feel that the PCA is not just a therapy based on theoretical ideas but more, as Rogers suggested, a 'way of being' (Rogers, 1980). There is a profound connection between one's sense of identity and approach. Identification with approach can be an intellectual one, but for many practitioners, it is deeply connected to how they experience themselves as people.

This sense of identification of approach with one's own fundamental experience of being is connected simultaneously with ethical values and philosophical positions. These values and positions are perceived as directly connected to particular approaches. Thus, approach and identity get seemingly inextricably linked. For some practitioners with particular interpretations of ethical-philosophical positions (e.g. Molyneux, 2014), parameters must be drawn and boundaries defended to preserve consistency and coherence of both personal and professional identity. Therefore, practitioners such as Molyneux (2014) perceive a 'problem with pluralism', since they perceive it as incoherent in terms of matching underlying philosophies to practice. This notion of some therapeutic approaches having a fundamental philosophical basis is also discussed in some literature (e.g. Tudor, 2018b). Other practitioners are more sceptical of these rationales for holding on tightly to particular positions/approaches.

It might be argued that 'adding on' and/or integration of other approaches/ techniques is inevitable to some degree, as the qualified practitioner will likely be exposed to other approaches throughout their career. Many practitioners will have experiences that lead to the discovery and practice of other approaches/techniques. This additional learning about – and perhaps practice of – other approaches/ techniques may or may not be seen by practitioners as meaning that their practice needs to be identified to either themselves or others as having changed from an original training/approach. Whether these kinds of changes are viewed as additions to practice or integrations of practice is subjective and, therefore, adds to the confusion around approach terminologies.

One post-qualification experience that might lead to a change in practice is working with specific client groups. For instance, in working with traumatised clients, technique-sceptical therapists might be expected to use psychoeducational techniques. This might leave the practitioner feeling uncomfortable in relation to – for example – the principles of the PCA. But then, if the experience of applying these techniques is perceived as helpful, an initially 'pure' practitioner might want to add or integrate them into their own practice.

Other practitioners not so attached to their approach in terms of identity might see the addition of techniques and ideas from other approaches as reflecting increased confidence over time. Trainees and newly qualified practitioners with less confidence might want to practise 'by the book' but over time develop the confidence to become more eclectic regarding what they offer clients. Practice might start with quite a narrow toolkit based on approach and identifying with that approach, but over time, if there are other tools to use in terms of techniques or theoretical lenses, then practice can become more flexible (see the next chapter for more on flexibility and rigidity).

Integrative versus Pluralistic Therapy

A large proportion of practitioners identify with the integrative approach (Hollanders & McLeod, 1999; McLeod, 2013), and an integrative approach to therapy, named as such, has been theorised and practised since the 1980s (Norcross & Saltzman, 1990). An integrative label does not necessarily mean integration of humanistic therapies exclusively (for instance, cognitive–analytic therapy is an integrative therapy), although, confusingly, integrative therapy is often associated with them.

The term 'pluralistic' applied to therapy is a relatively recent development and still relatively unknown and unused compared to 'integrative', especially in the USA and other countries. Although there are significant differences in meaning between integrative and pluralistic, some might perceive that these differences do not exist – or, if they do exist, they have not been theoretically or practically adhered to in the evolution of pluralistic therapy. It could be said that both the theoreticians and practitioners of pluralistic therapy have not adequately differentiated themselves from the integrative umbrella. Indeed, three factors that Norcross and Saltzman (1990) perceived, more than thirty years ago, to be causes of the interest in integration were:

1   The proliferation of brand-name therapies, leading to fragmentation, a deafening cacophony of rival claims, and excessive choice
2   The nascent consensus that no one approach is clinically adequate for all problems, patients, and situations
3   The equality of therapeutic outcomes, with some exceptions, ascribed to empirically evaluated therapies

(1990, p. 3)

These factors are noticeably similar to what Cooper and McLeod (e.g. 2011) use as central arguments for their more recent pluralistic therapy, discussed specifically as an approach and identity in a later section. In the literature, Cooper and McLeod (e.g. 2011) have attempted to differentiate pluralistic approaches to therapy but have also referred to their framework as being a 'meta-model of therapy integration' (McLeod & Sundet, 2016, p. 160). They acknowledge the pluralistic aspects of both integrative and eclectic approaches but reiterate that it is only in their pluralistic approach that collaboration is central – in other words, they are suggesting that therapists can be integrative or eclectic but not involve clients in decision-making about therapeutic methods. They also more explicitly acknowledge that their approach is informed by 'humanistic, person-centred and postmodern values', while claiming that it also 'aims to ... embrace ... the whole range of effective therapeutic methods and concepts' (Cooper & McLeod, 2011, p. 11).

From a pluralistic perspective, most practitioners, even if they prefer a more purist approach to therapy in terms of their own practice, might support a more pluralistic provision of therapy at organisational levels. Pluralism as a philosophy and a political ideology can underlie a push for more pluralistic provision, which includes integrative and pluralistic therapy, without needing to proselytise for integrative or pluralistic therapies per se.

Newer Approaches/Identities

In more recent years, in parallel with broader political developments, there have been an increasing number of therapeutic identities based on social identities and intersectionalities (as discussed in the previous chapter). Often, contemporary therapists identify with and/or identify their therapeutic practices as being supportive or affirmative of, for instance, neurodiversity; gender nonconformity; disability; different racial, religious, and ethnic groups; and other intersections. Pluralism itself is often seen as synonymous with multiculturalism, although in this book the meanings of pluralism go far wider than that relatively narrow meaning, as discussed previously.

Pluralistic Therapy as an Identity and Approach

In this book, I often refer to pluralistic 'approaches', 'perspectives', and 'practices' because I see pluralism as something that is not 'owned' by Cooper and McLeod; simultaneously, I do recognise that when practitioners refer to 'pluralistic therapy' they are usually referring to Cooper and McLeod's framework.

The relationship between pluralistic therapy as a practice and pluralism as a philosophy/perspective is of central importance, and, to a certain extent, they are inextricably linked. However, for me, the meaning of pluralism in therapy goes deeper and wider than the framework Cooper, McLeod, and others have devised. Arguably, Mick Cooper and John McLeod's articulation of a pluralistic therapy is not actually pluralistic, as attempting to define what pluralistic therapy is and how it should be practised inevitably closes down options. However, their ambition for a pluralistic therapy to be open to external examination by, for instance, membership bodies and standardised research protocols is understandable. Otherwise, pluralism remains more elusive in terms of being able to prove itself to potentially interested stakeholders. I contend that pluralism is something that has always existed in therapy and is more useful as a philosophical position which can inform therapists and therapy providers rather than needing to be a named approach as such.

Self-defined pluralistic practitioners draw upon different approaches and techniques, either for different clients or for the same client. They do not perceive pragmatic, ethical, or philosophical problems with this. Other practitioners do perceive those kinds of problems, so they are more hesitant to embrace pluralistic ideas for their own practices.

There is the possibility of holding a vision for therapy in which practitioners are not pluralistic in their own individual practice but, from a pluralistic perspective, welcome the prospect of clients being able to choose from an array of therapies and appreciate the value of most therapeutic approaches for different clients at different times. At this level, the issue of whether pluralistic therapy in itself is beneficial for clients is not of concern, but rather whether clients should or should not be allowed easier access to and movement between different approaches and be encouraged in these choices by therapists and therapy providers. This would reflect the view that different therapies are better for different levels of personal development and development within the therapy process (e.g. Marquis, 2008; Wilber, 2000). This view also suggests that attempting to practise with a particular therapeutic approach with a client whose level of development does not match the level at which the therapy is aimed can be counter-therapeutic or ineffective. This might be one explanation for high drop-out rates, for instance, as occurs in the UK's CBT-dominated IAPT programme (e.g. Kelly & Moloney, 2018).

As a counter-argument to the idea that therapy is best practised from one philosophical position and/or approach, it might be suggested that therapists who are not eclectic are potentially practising unethically, since if therapists are not doing all that they can with all that they know, whether that is a part of their approach or not, then that is unethical practice.

Maybe the majority of therapists practise pluralistically, in any case. Research by Thoma and Cecero (2009) supports the idea that most therapists are pluralistic. They surveyed 209 therapists and found that therapists actually used more techniques from outside their identified approach than from within it.

Overall, for me, pluralism, as stated previously, is not so much a separate approach but rather a dimension that runs through all therapies and therapists. This dimension is sometimes absent, sometimes present, sometimes overt, sometimes covert, sometimes consciously applied or integrated into an individual's practice in a way that the practitioner feels no need to name it as such; an automatic, learned-from-experience approach, not that special, just how therapists work with the client who 'comes in'. Practitioners who bring everything they have to work with the client will inevitably practise pluralistically because they have learnt from a diverse array of sources.

A pluralistic attitude, or an explicit articulation of a pluralistic approach (such as the pluralistic therapy framework), offers hope for some practitioners who practise pluralistically that their identity and approach might be more highly valued. Other practitioners fear pluralism might efface legitimate and valuable differences between approaches and discount the importance of understanding and responding to philosophical positions underlying single-model approaches.

Concluding Thoughts

In conclusion, therapeutic approaches are often deeply intertwined with therapist identities. Although this is not always the case – some therapists are more relaxed about practising without needing to identify with particular approaches – when it comes to the issue of whether therapists should be more or less pluralistic in their practices, the approach/identity interface is crucial. How practitioners respond to the idea of therapy becoming more informed by pluralism, philosophically and/or pragmatically, reflects various felt positions in relation to therapeutic approaches and identities.

Chapter 6

Flexibility and Rigidity

Flexibility in Cooper et al.'s Pluralistic Therapy

Flexibility in 'methods' is probably what most professionals and laypersons assume to be the main feature of a pluralistic practice. Cooper and McLeod (2007) draw upon an example of a bereaved person to illustrate how different approaches have different methods to work with such a client. They explain that a pluralistic practitioner would discuss the different methods they could use with the client before prescribing any methods from within a solitary model. This collaboration with the client about how they want to work, rather than assuming the methods of the practitioner's preferred model are needed and wanted, is a central feature of their pluralistic practice. There is also an emphasis on client choice rather than the client being allocated to a therapeutic approach without consultation and information-giving – a relatively normal occurrence outside private practice.

It is sometimes confusing as to whether pluralistic therapy wants to be a distinctive approach (e.g. McLeod, 2018) or a framework. I prefer the latter conceptualisation, as that allows it an open flexibility with the potential to be more genuinely pluralistic in contrast to setting out protocols such as goals, tasks, and methods (e.g. Brown & Smith, 2023).

However, leaving aside the issue of whether pluralistic therapy is an approach or a framework, the importance of flexibility in any practice proclaiming itself to be pluralistic is central. As Brown and Smith put it: '[t]here are multiple ways that a client can experience problems in living ... [t]o respond to this, the pluralistic framework serves to structure flexibility into therapy' (2023, p. 4). They suggest that flexibility is one of the 'fundamental principles that guide pluralistic therapy' (p. 20), and this can operate in several domains, including 'the structure, process, communication style or platform, and characteristics of the relationship' (p. 24). For instance, in terms of platform, some clients might want to vary between in-person, video, telephone, and text (Smith & de la Prida, 2021; see also McLeod, 2018). From a pluralistic perspective, if the therapist has the skills to manage this, then such flexibility is possible. Brown and Smith (2023) also point out that this flexibility needs to be ongoing throughout the therapy.

DOI: 10.4324/9781003468332-6

In this spirit, pluralistic practice can be accused of encouraging therapists to be 'therapeutic Jacks of all trades and masters of none' (Grant, 2015). Cooper and McLeod's recommendation is that therapists should not practise outside of their competence: if, through collaborative metacommunication about therapeutic methods, it is concluded that the way the client wants to work cannot be offered at a competent level by the therapist, then the pluralistic solution would be to refer that client on, or for the therapist to educate/train him- or herself to a sufficient level of competence, assuming that to be practicable (see also Brown & Smith, 2023).

Pluralistic therapy is a 'relatively new approach' that its proselytisers characterise as 'offering *flexible* [my italics], collaborative forms of help to our clients and service users' (Abertay University, 2018). In my view, there is not a strict either/or divide between those who practise pluralistically and those who do not; rather, there is a continuum of practice from strictly fixed singular approaches to flexible multiple approaches.

The Flexibility–Rigidity Continuum

From a feminist or Jungian perspective, flexibility in therapeutic practice might be seen as a 'feminine' quality versus the demand for more 'masculine' precision in work and professional environments. In a patriarchal society, this precision might be overvalued as a useful element in therapy in comparison to flexibility. Rizq, following Derrida, characterises work cultures, particularly within NPM cultures, as encouraging a 'phallogocentric' attitude to caring versus the 'emotional, messy – and maternal – aspects of caregiving' (Rizq, 2016, p. 79) in which a more flexible, adaptive approach might be a more pragmatic response to those suffering with personal distress.

It is unlikely that any therapist is completely flexible or completely rigid in their practice. Therefore, it is helpful to conceive the variability of therapists and therapies in terms of their flexibility and rigidity as a continuum in which practitioners locate themselves more towards one end than the other.

Horses for Courses versus One Size Fits All

As the saying goes, there are 'different horses for different courses'. The basis of pluralism as applied to therapy is the belief that different clients need different things at different times. This belief is shared by many therapists, whether or not they identify themselves as being pluralistic. Conversely, advocating for the rightness and exclusiveness of one's own single-approach practice implies a 'one-size-fits-all' attitude. This variation of attitude amongst practitioners between a more casual 'horses for courses' versus 'one size fits all' is a significant cause of professional arguments about pluralistic perspectives and/or practices.

As discussed in the previous chapter about therapeutic approaches and identities, it is possible to be very flexible even within an approach identified as singular. For instance, the PCA – because it attempts to be client-led, emphasising the client's exploration towards their own understandings and encouraging their own meaning-making and decision-making – has more potential to go in a multitude of directions: the PCA therapist is less likely to shut down explorations by taking over the direction of the process. Regarding how person-centred therapists respond to their clients, it might be argued that as long as the response is empathic and non-judgmental that is the 'intervention'. Despite its sometimes strict adherence to the 'core conditions' (e.g. Mearns et al., 2013), the PCA is, in practice, highly flexible. Transactional Analysis (TA), while having a comprehensive theory and highly developed protocols of practice, is flexible in a slightly different way by being fully open to the influence of other perspectives such as postmodernism and existentialism (e.g. Erskine, 2010). Practitioners identifying with various singular approaches often see the value of being flexible not just within their approach but, sometimes, by 'borrowing' from other approaches.

This practitioner flexibility challenges the rationale of providers who respond to RCTs and the underlying assumption that practitioners do adhere to strict implementations of their approach (McLeod, 2013). Also, in practice, therapists often have a variety of job roles, so it is not unusual, for instance, for someone trained in CBT to also be identified as a generic 'counsellor' in some contexts. In those contexts, when other things are demanded of them by the providers and the clients, they are likely to be more flexible.

In contemporary therapeutic practices, many practitioners who identify as belonging to a single approach have become enamoured of teaching clients practices such as mindfulness, breathing techniques, and visualisations. And most practitioners are flexible enough to add on or integrate such practices without much ado.

Therapists can often find being more flexible as personally liberating by not feeling too bound up in a particular way of doing things. Ultimately, it is likely that experienced therapists understand that the more they can bring of themselves to the process the better, and flexibility enables them to be more themselves rather than adhering strictly to the 'rules' of any given approach. Thinking that one has to say and do things in particular ways goes against the notion of what Rogers called therapist congruence (e.g. Mearns et al., 2013).

However, also within the PCA, some practitioners feel that their approach is inherently different from other approaches in its commitment to what it offers and its belief in people. The central belief is that the PCA is based solely on the relationship in a profoundly and philosophically different way from other approaches. With such an attitude, it is perhaps not surprising that some of the more impassioned critiques of pluralistic therapy have come from the person-centred community (e.g. Ong et al., 2020). For PCA therapists sharing these interpretations of what the PCA means for practice, it is simply not possible to bring in other approaches/techniques if the therapist has a proper understanding and commitment to the PCA.

For some practitioners, flexibility might be based on the presenting symptoms. So, if the client is recently bereaved, then it makes sense to work more closely with the core conditions and stay with the client's process as much as possible. On the other hand, symptoms such as anxiety and stress can respond well to CBT techniques, which challenge overly negative thinking and can be worked with in the client's everyday lives through homework such as daily thought records and recognition of 'thinking errors'. Therapists often use the metaphor of having a 'toolbox' (ideas and techniques they have picked up via training, supervision, practice, and CPD). On that basis, these tools for the work only need a pragmatic rather than a theoretical or philosophical rationale (e.g. Carrell, 2001). Brown and Smith (2023) suggest that 'having a toolkit from which to offer clients a choice in the way they think therapy should be done is essential in pluralistic practice' (p. 215).

Pluralistic perspectives and practices have as a central concern the danger of therapy practice becoming inflexible: 'Practicing pluralistically means accepting each client, negotiating ways of working with them and rejecting the notion that one size fits all' (Thompson & Cooper, 2012, p. 65). There is supporting evidence that flexible ways of working (rather than strict adherence to particular protocols) improve outcomes (e.g. Owen & Hilsenroth, 2014).

However, the privileging of large-scale quantitative research (e.g. RCTs) by public health bodies and other stakeholders has ultimately led to a 'one-size-fits-all' culture in which clients have little choice beyond a narrow band of 'evidence-based' therapies. The need for an apparently unified therapy (as discussed in the previous chapter) to be rigidly adhered to at the point of evidence-gathering (at least the kind of evidence that counts for such bodies) puts practices and practitioners who are more flexible at an obvious disadvantage, at least within the public sector. The impact of this inflexibility on clients also cannot be understated: therapist inflexibility in relation to clients in terms of the imposition of goals, methods, and techniques can all potentially harm rather than help clients (Curran et al., 2019; Norcross & Wampold, 2018; Smith & de la Prida, 2021). Conversely, some evidence suggests that clients prefer therapists to be flexible, and this flexibility can lead to improved outcomes (Cooper & McLeod, 2011).

Third-sector agencies such as Mind (2013) have criticised the NHS's Talking Therapies (TT) service (previously IAPT) – which, in any case, only targets two diagnoses (anxiety and depression) – for its inflexibility in providing therapy. It does not serve black and ethnic minority communities as much as other communities and does not deal 'with issues of culture, class and systemic oppression' (Boyles & Fathi, 2019, p. 246). A participant in Boyles and Fathi's (2019) research is quoted as saying: 'We need services in the community, we need creativity and flexibility in our model'. These qualities of creativity and flexibility are sadly lacking in public sector therapy provision.

Cooper and McLeod (2011) suggest a pluralistic model for the provision of therapy services might be flexible in terms of offering choices to clients about:

> frequency of sessions … length of sessions … choice of therapist … access to the therapist other than in face-to-face meetings … capacity to change therapist, or to see more than one therapist at the same time … availability of couple, family and group work … availability of self-help resources … access to specialist treatments … location of therapy.
>
> (p. 150)

This is the kind of service and services therapists can offer in a world not so enslaved by self-defeating audit systems usually geared to providing fewer options rather than more. It might be argued that this pluralistic ideal for therapy would be too expensive for public sector provision, but if outcomes were to be more effective, then it might be that shutting down options rather than increasing them is a false economy (see Carey, 2005 and Carey & Mullan, 2007 cited in Cooper & McLeod, 2011).

Professionalisation and Regulation

It has also been argued that professionalisation and regulation encourage therapists to stay in their box (Morgan-Ayrs, 2016). Pluralism has the potential to free therapeutic practice from box-containing and box-ticking cultures. The appeal of practising in a 'box without walls', as one therapist I know put it, is that it would allow practice to be flexible, a prerequisite of any pluralistic practice. Over-regulation of therapeutic practices could lead to (if it has not already done so) unnecessary demarcation of approaches and practices akin to over-zealous demarcation of job roles. There is also the danger, which has already begun to manifest, that therapists who do not choose to use empirically supported treatments or evidence-based practice will be accused of being 'unethical' (e.g., see Goodman, 2016, p. 79).

Therapists sympathetic to a pluralistic approach to therapy have a flexible framework and attitude towards practice, rooted in an awareness of the client's needs and their own skills and competence to make different kinds of interventions.

Flexibility and the Relationship

One belief which lends itself to a more flexible attitude to practice is that 'it's the relationship' which is the most important component of effective therapeutic practice. In this view, the relationship potentially trumps all other components of therapeutic efficacy; therefore, as long as the relationship is working, then 'whatever works' within the relationship, whether that be a different approach or technique, is for the good. The importance of the relationship in therapeutic practice forms the basis of exploration in the next chapter.

Chapter 7

It's the Relationship, Stupid

Petruska Clarkson's *The Therapeutic Relationship* (2003/1995) offered a frame-work based on the 'relationship', which, according to Clarkson, is the 'factor' which is 'vivid and obvious as the substructure in which most psychotherapies find their being' (p. xvi). In the foreword to the second edition, Christopher Hauke describes the book as:

> a postmodern text that is clearly comfortable with the *pluralism* [my italics] "universes of discourse" that exist in psychology and psychotherapy today, and which require of us a tolerance and a revaluation of fragmentation, a fresh look at old essentialisms. What is "right" in psychology is what is right in each par-ticular context, person or treatment. Clarkson's book helps us to track the many contours of psychotherapeutic practice in a way which avoids hierarchies, val-ues subjectivity and a choice of paths ...
>
> (Hauke, 2003/1995, p. xiii)

In this passage, Hauke, in addition to referring to pluralism directly, also points to her framework as encouraging qualities and values in therapeutic practice, which will come to be similarly evoked by pluralistic therapy theorists several years later.

Clarkson herself, in the preface to the second edition, states her five-relationship model

> provides a framework for integrating *pluralism* [my italics] or deepening sin-gularity using a framework of *five* [italics in original] facets of relationship potentially available in *every* [italics in original] kind of counselling or psycho-dynamic work. And in all professions. And in all of life ...
>
> (Clarkson, 2003/1995, p. xxvii)

Her wish to 'integrate' pluralism reflects what, in my view, is confusion and con-flation between pluralism and integration, as discussed in previous chapters. In-deed, Clarkson's model was the basis for many 'integrative' courses; however, although Clarkson identified it as 'integrative', her model can be seen as having foundations that align with a pluralistic view of therapy. Since the conflation and

DOI: 10.4324/9781003468332-7

confusion between 'integrative' and 'pluralistic' has become so pervasive and entrenched, it might be more helpful to think of the variety of integrative therapies as more or less pluralistic, with some integrative therapies not pluralistic at all. Clarkson's model has the ambition for a unitary framework while allowing for a plurality of therapies to flourish within it. This is quite different from versions of 'integrative' therapy moving towards, for instance, ideals of a more genericised, 'evidence-based' psychotherapy, somehow transcending, but not including, established therapeutic orientations coming from psychodynamic, humanistic, and other approaches.

For the purposes of this chapter, leaving aside further analysis of similarities and differences between integration and pluralism, to previous and subsequent chapters, her analyses and definitions of the *therapeutic relationship* point to what I intend 'the relationship' to mean when I say, only half-jokingly, 'it's the relationship, stupid'. I intend the relationship to mean all five facets which Clarkson elucidates: I am not merely referring to the working alliance or a relationally deep 'I-Thou' encounter. It is the quality of the relationship, yes, but also using the relationship and being aware of what is going on in it, as articulated clearly and comprehensively by Clarkson.

She suggests that the five different 'facets' of relationship that can all be useful to different clients at different times are: 1) the working alliance, 2) the transference/countertransference relationship, 3) the developmentally needed or reparative relationship, 4) the person-to-person or dialogic relationship, and 5) the transpersonal relationship. From a pluralistic perspective, what is liberating for therapists about this framework is that it implies that it is always the relationship and the type of relationship which is most important *in any therapeutic process* over and above named approaches and specific techniques.

As Clarkson states: 'the bulk of the research points to the fact that the most important factor in effective psychotherapeutic work is the relationship between the client and the counsellor' (Clarkson, 2003/1995, p. xvi). Richard Erskine concurs that the 'therapeutic relationship itself is the counselor's and psychotherapist's most powerful intervention' (Erskine & Moursund, 2022, p. xx; see also Norcross & Lambert, 2019).

Additionally, and importantly, as we begin to think about the future of therapy (to be discussed specifically in the final chapter), this framework ensures therapy is kept in the realm of the *human*. As computing and AI technologies advance, the therapy field finds itself threatened by automated therapy derived from massive data sets. Elizabeth Cotton has described this process as one aspect of an 'uberisation' of therapy (Cotton, 2021). One major professional body, the National Counselling and Psychotherapy Society (NCPS), has allied with a major awarding body, the Counselling and Psychotherapy Central Awarding Body (CPCAB), to campaign for therapeutic relationships as a 'human connection' in response to the increasing number of digital therapy apps and AI therapist chatbots (NCPS, 2024). Yet, if therapy can be defined as something which does not really exist unless it takes place within a human relationship, then there will be room for computerised and AI versions of therapy without them being mistaken for therapy itself. The more technical and technicist therapies have the most to lose here, but even CBT, perhaps more vulnerable to these technological changes, as long as it insists on a relational dimension, can ensure its place in the realm of human-based practice.

Research, the Medical Model, and Pluralism

Seemingly simple relational qualities are central to effective therapy. However, these relational qualities are often overlooked when researchers seek to identify what makes therapy effective and efficient. Research, which providers take seriously, attempts to ignore the relationship by trying to not let it confound other variables (usually named approaches). Thus, researchers often purposefully exclude therapeutic factors which are, for instance, 'common … extratherapeutic … [or] placebo' (Reeves, 2014). RCTs and other nomothetic research methods reflect 'wide ranging and fundamental methodological flaws for establishing effective treatment' (Thornton, 2018). These fundamental flaws have devastating real-world effects because they often lead to a monistic 'one-size-fits-all' provision of therapy, resulting in less choice for clients and less chance of clients gaining relief from their suffering (SPR, 2022).

Therapists and therapies that either support or integrate more easily with scientistic medical models can be seen as valuing an 'instrumental' approach, and these approaches are the approaches which tend to be favoured by institutions insisting on 'evidence-based' or 'empirically supported' treatments. Meanwhile, humanistic and person-centred approaches – which might be seen as more 'relational' and valorising the power of the relationship as the central component of effective therapy – are marginalised because, in effect, their philosophical and psychological assumptions and foundations are not understood or recognised by those instigating and investigating the research. This important distinction between 'instrumental' and 'relational' approaches can be explored in more depth in Rowan (2016).

The pluralistic framework can be viewed as a kind of polite fight-back for an array of therapies which were getting 'lost' not just in the 'therapy wars' (Saltzman & Norcross, 1990) but also in the 'research wars'. The main line of attack on 'evidence-based practice and empirically supported treatment movements' was that the factors of therapeutic effectiveness which therapists themselves believe to be important – namely the variables of the therapist, the relationship, and 'other common factors' – were effectively ignored by this kind of research (Wampold & Bhati, 2004).

However, Norcross and Lambert (2019) warn against conceptualising a 'false dichotomy of method versus relationship', especially since it has led to and continues to advance what they consider to be a 'pernicious and insidious … polarizing effect on the discipline [of therapy]' (p. 1). They characterise this polarising effect as reflecting the 'culture wars in psychotherapy'. This aligns with my sense that these wars have some roots in profoundly differing ontological worldviews of a materialist, scientistic mainstream culture versus a more transpersonal/spiritual *counter* culture which brought its own ideas and practices to the world of therapy from the 1960s onwards. These themes will be developed in more detail in the next chapter 'Therapy Wars'.

CBT and the Relationship

In recent years, there has been a hegemonic rise of CBT, which has marginalised more traditional and more 'relational' therapies – humanistic and psychodynamic therapies, in particular (e.g. Barkham et al., 2017).

In 1979, *Cognitive Therapy of Depression*, the first 'treatment manual' which describes not only how to practise a particular approach but also how to practise that approach to treat a particular disorder, was published (Beck et al., 1979). This manual was produced by the proponents of cognitive therapy. Cognitive therapy would later be the basis for CBT and could be seen as the first RCT-friendly treatment that could easily provide the kind of medicalised research comfortable with providing treatments for symptoms – as opposed to therapeutic relationships for people – that was, and still is, favoured by medical providers.

The PCA, Integrative Therapy, and the Relationship

In contrast, the PCA is based on a fundamental belief in the relationship and the relationship alone as the healing, therapeutic factor. From a person-centred perspective, the main factors that enable the therapist to co-create a therapeutic relationship are unconditional positive regard, empathy, and genuineness – the latter sometimes called congruence. These three (initially six) are commonly known as the 'core conditions' (e.g. Mearns et al., 2013).

Rogers is famous for this quote about therapy:

> …in my early professional years I was asking the question, How can I treat, or cure, or change this person? Now I would phrase the question in this way: How can I provide a relationship which this person may use for his own personal growth?
>
> (Rogers, 1961, p. 32)

While many therapeutic approaches align with a relational emphasis, the PCA, with Rogers's seminal texts, can lay claim, more than most, historically and currently, to focusing on the relationship as the central component of meaningful therapy. Rogers states that his hypothesis about the relationship is: If I can provide a certain type of relationship, the other person will discover within himself the capacity to use that relationship for growth and change and personal development will occur (1961, p. 33).

The 'certain type of relationship' is one characterised by the core conditions. Rogers asserted that '[n]o other conditions are necessary' and that they are 'sufficient' (Rogers, 1957, p. 96). The debate as to whether that statement is true or whether clients need more is one which continues and forms one of many splits in the profession. It is one of multiple issues in what has been characterised as the 'therapy wars' (Saltzman & Norcross, 1990), again to be discussed more fully in the next chapter.

Erskine (Erskine & Moursund, 2022), similarly, framing his approach as 'integrative', identifies empathy as the 'key element in the therapeutic relationship' (p. xix). The communication of this empathic understanding being conveyed to the client, also emphasised in the PCA (e.g. Mearns et al., 2013), he names as 'contact-in-relationship' (p. xix) and says that this communication is 'beyond empathy'. For the therapeutic relationship to be effective and go beyond empathy (as Erskine articulates it), the therapists must bring 'attunement, inquiry and involvement' (Erskine & Moursund, 2022) to the process. Attunement is demonstrated by the therapist resonating accurately with 'what the client presents'; inquiry implies 'not only questions' but is 'woven into every response that invites the client to deepen his own awareness of his own internal process'; and involvement reflects the 'therapist's commitment to being an active, caring, vulnerable, and authentic participant in the therapeutic process' (2022). Most therapeutic approaches would encourage these qualities – even if they do not use person-centred or integrative terminology – and certainly most humanistic therapies, if not all psychodynamic and cognitive approaches, would do likewise. These qualities are also encouraged in pluralistic therapy, which will be discussed in the next section.

Pluralism, Pluralistic Therapy, and the Relationship

The valuing of both client and therapist perspectives is central to Cooper and McLeod's pluralistic practice and leads to their particular emphasis for it to have a 'collaborative relationship' at its 'heart' (Cooper & McLeod, 2007, p. 139). In this regard, pluralistic practice seems to be an attempt to maximise the benefit of the 'working alliance' and the 'therapeutic relationship' (Clarkson, 2003/1995), which many researchers and practitioners see as a key factor in therapeutic effectiveness (e.g. Fluckiger et al., 2018; Horvath & Greenberg, 1994). Cooper and McLeod (2007) cite further research evidence (e.g. Addis & Jacobson, 2000) to support their view that the collaborative qualities they associate with pluralistic therapy improve outcomes.

It might be that the controversial 'dodo verdict' about therapeutic approaches has been reached *because* 'it's the relationship' (see Bohart, 2000; Gilbert & Orlans, 2011). Maybe this verdict exists because it is not different kinds of approaches which make any significant difference. If it is the relationship that differentiates therapeutic effectiveness, then that effectiveness is more likely to be caused by client factors, therapist factors, and relationship factors in the interplay between clients and therapists: the dodo verdict exists because so many researchers have their eye on the wrong variable. This is a common theme in the literature about therapy research, and although this is well known and commonly discussed, most researchers and commissioning bodies still insist on comparing therapeutic approaches over other variables.

However, the Cooper and McLeod framework/approach does seem to have an instrumental emphasis. The most apparent manifestation of this is that the framework centres the envisaged collaborative relationship between therapists and clients on the 'goals, tasks and methods of therapy' (Cooper & McLeod, 2011, p. 27). It might be that, in practice, loose interpretations of these terms leaves enough leeway for less clinical applications, but the use of them leaves the impression of an overly rational attitude to the therapeutic relationship. Interestingly, in more recent years, Cooper has talked more about 'directionality' than goals, perhaps partly as a response to those who struggle with the utilitarian language of the framework (Cooper, 2019a). Although Cooper and McLeod say they value therapies that might be characterised as more 'relational', their approach often comes across as describing an approach that is more about 'doing' than 'being'. Their wish for pluralism to be seen as pragmatic and tangible necessarily devalues approaches that might be seen as idealistic and which value more intangible aspects of the therapeutic relationship as a healing process.

Being versus Doing

For some practitioners, especially those with more existential or transpersonal inclinations, the importance and centrality of the relationship in and for therapy also reflects prioritising a philosophical position of valuing 'being' over the more usual privileging of 'doing' in contemporary life (e.g. Rowan, 2005a). In the therapy context, this specifically refers to the valuing of being *with* clients over doing *to* clients.

In relation to Cooper and McLeod's pluralistic therapy, the concept of 'tasks' as a necessary component of therapy can seem like a 'doing to' rather than a 'being with'. Similarly, the word 'toolkit', which some therapists use – and Brown and Smith (2023) describe as 'essential' for pluralistic practice (p. 215) – to describe drawing on different techniques can seem like it is going away from the idea of therapy as a relational process into more of an instrumental activity.

In general, the assumption that therapy is first and foremost described best by approach implies that the most important thing about therapy is what it *does* rather than what it *is*. This may seem unnecessarily pedantic, but I suggest actually – and especially from a pluralistic perspective – that the implications are profound. For instance, the routine division of therapies into a 'big four' (i.e. psychodynamic, humanistic, integrative, cognitive-behavioural – see, for example, Dryden, 1999) implicitly encourages an understanding of therapy as a 'doing' activity rather than a 'being with' relationship. The taken-for-granted assumptions behind conceptions of therapy practice as fitting into labels take the focus away from the personal and individual 'being' of therap*ists* towards the depersonalised and organisational 'doing' of therap*ies*. This, in itself, potentially encourages a monistic rather than a pluralistic understanding of what therapy has to offer.

This emphasis on the 'being' as well as the 'doing' of therapy has been especially articulated in the literature coming out of humanistic therapy (e.g. Rowan, 2016). Yalom has also referred to the importance of 'presence' and how therapists, through anxiety and restlessness, can be easily distracted by trying to 'do' therapy rather than paying full attention to the client in a 'being' mode (e.g. Yalom, 2015). The notion of 'presence' is intangible and elusive, so it is difficult to measure or monitor; however, its importance is central to the therapeutic enterprise. The incommensurability between what might be important about therapy and what can realistically be researched is a major problem.

Concluding Thoughts

Overall, it is a common belief of therapists that it is the relationship – rather than techniques – which is the most important factor in therapeutic effectiveness; unconditional positive regard, for example, has been found to be more important than any technique (e.g. Farber & Doolin, 2011). There is quite substantial theoretical support (e.g. Middleton, 2015; Norcross, 2011; Pilgrim et al., 2009) and empirical data behind the assumption of the therapeutic relationship as central to the beneficial processes and outcomes of all therapies (e.g. Norcross & Goldfried, 1992; Norcross & Lambert, 2011a; 2011b). This research is widely known and discussed within the therapy professions.

However, the belief in the primacy of the relationship is not shared by all: narrative therapists, for instance, emphasise the distressed person's relationships in everyday life, as opposed to the constructed view of the therapist–client relationship as central (Sundet & McLeod, 2016). Research also suggests that although the relationship has a more significant effect on outcome than the treatment method it is still far less than 'patient contribution' (e.g. Norcross & Lambert, 2011a; 2011b). It has been suggested that clients contribute to positive outcomes, for example, by helping to build and maintain a therapeutic alliance and sustaining a belief that therapy will be helpful (e.g. Bohart & Tallman, 1999; Sparks & Duncan, 2016). Significantly, in relation to pluralism, it is suggested that, amongst other factors, it is 'the client's preferences for intervention that drive therapy' (Sparks & Duncan, 2016, p. 72).

The emphasis on the importance of the relationship connects to generic personal factors such as warmth, rapport, being kind, being gentle, and listening as at the core of effective therapy rather than any particular approach. If, on the whole then, therapists themselves do not conceptualise different approaches as that central to effectiveness, it is no wonder that they might be frustrated by the dubious basis of research which insists on attempting to compare approaches rather than the qualities of the therapists delivering those approaches. This is another important issue in the debates around pluralism and purism: it is not just that respect for a variety of approaches is being called for. Additionally, it is that focusing on the title or label of a particular approach fundamentally misses what might be important about those approaches in terms of their underlying processes (e.g. Gilbert & Orlans, 2011; Norcross, 2002).

The common catchphrase by therapists that 'it's the relationship', while having substantial support from the research, simultaneously suffers from a seeming vagueness, which allows therapists and therapies that seem to 'do' more to gain advantage. It is easier for commissioners of services to understand and support therapies that pursue an instrumental rather than a relational approach. Practitioners have a grasp of 'the relationship' being an essential aspect of therapy, but the elusive nature of what this actually means leads to technique-based therapies being more favoured. This is another example of gaps between the personal yet empirical evidence of an individual's practice in particular (pluralistic) as opposed to generalised evidence from the whole (monistic).

I would suggest that a major long-term aim of the pluralistic agenda is to re-incorporate therapists and therapies which emphasise the importance of relational factors (both humanistic and psychodynamic approaches) into the public sector by re-translating these kinds of factors into instrumental language that can be measured and understood by the gatekeepers of provision. Some professionals perceive this agenda and project as urgent (e.g. Ingersoll, 2008; Loewenthal, 2016) if 'traditional' therapies are to survive. Ultimately, however, therapy is a socially constructed activity that cannot be reduced from idiosyncratic encounters between human beings and is inherently uncertain and unpredictable – almost the quintessence of what science cannot capture: the multitudinous variables of a human relationship.

Finally, it is worth contemplating the words of Krishnamurti: 'Action has meaning only in relationship and without understanding relationship, action on any level will only breed conflict. The understanding of relationship is infinitely more important than the search for any plan of action ...' (Krishnamurti quoted in Mate, 2019, epigraph).

Chapter 8

Therapy Wars

A Brief History of the Medical Model and Scientism in Therapy

In 1859, 'The Boston School of Psychopathology' was founded. William James, an important figure both for psychology and pluralism, joined this group, which became the 'epicenter of the new talk therapy' (Wampold & Imel, 2015, p. 17). The group was important in the long term for beginning to establish talking therapies in the USA as a legitimate medical/scientific activity. The wish for scientific and/or medical credibility for therapy by interested groups is deeply rooted. It might be argued that the pluralism of therapy begins at this stage, when potential conflicts can be seen to emerge between newer, medicalised, scientific versions of therapy and earlier, non-medicalised, intuitive, 'spiritual' or 'artistic' versions of therapy, situated in a historical context where it seems these apparent opposites are irreconcilable (Wampold & Imel, 2015).

A scientific drive in psychology runs throughout its history and has led to the contemporary prominence of 'evidence-based therapies'. A similar and related drive to 'medicalise' therapy has deep roots: James was himself trained in medicine (Wampold & Imel, 2015). At first, the medical profession was confused by a practice that used a non-medical intervention (i.e. 'talk'), but it would come to claim this practice as its own. In 1894, James himself urged 'medicine' to study and ascertain the laws of 'mental therapeutics' (2015). Only a few years earlier Van Renterghem and Van Eeden had been the first physicians to label themselves as 'psychotherapists' and 'opened a clinic of Suggestive Psychotherapy in Amsterdam in 1887' (McLeod, 2013, p. 22). This wish to associate talking therapies with medicine was, arguably, motivated by a need and desire to gain status not so easily accomplished in other disciplines.

The publication by Sigmund Freud of *The Interpretation of Dreams* in 1900 marked the beginning of psychoanalysis as a nascent theory, as opposed to just a practice. He took his psychoanalytic ideas to America in 1909 via a series of lectures at Clark University, where he also met and talked with James. Wampold and Imel (2015) state that '[w]ithin six years psychoanalysis had become the predominant form of psychotherapy in the United States' (p. 18). If Freudian psychoanalysis

DOI: 10.4324/9781003468332-8

might have been a unified idea and profession, as Freud initially hoped for (see, e.g., Ekins & Freeman, 1994), it was already splitting by this time due to the personal and theoretical arguments developing between Freud, Joseph Breuer, Alfred Adler, and Carl Jung. Thus, in 1911, Adler introduced 'individual psychology', and by 1913 Jung was working out 'analytic psychology'; so, an originally unified school of psychoanalysis was already developing pluralities of thought and practice. It is also notable that a major reason Jung split from Freud was because Freud dismissed the importance of religion and spirituality, aspects of what has become known as the 'transpersonal' (e.g. Rowan, 2005a): Jung laid the foundations for the many different types of transpersonal therapies which were to emerge from that point onward.

In the 1920s, the relative simplicity of splits within a psychoanalytic, cognitive, and emotional model of therapy began to be challenged by the rise of behaviourism, which was 'openly disdainful' (Wampold & Imel, 2015, p. 20) of Freudian theory. This intensified the desire of various theorists and practitioners to be 'better' than their contemporaries or forebears. The behaviourists, especially, wanted to claim a superior scientific status, hence their focus on behaviour – which can allegedly be objectively observed, as opposed to thoughts and feelings, which are inherently subjective and open to dispute and interpretation.

The competitiveness between these different approaches, and their assertions of superiority, was challenged as nonsensical and invalid as early as 1936, with the publication of Saul Rosenzweig's paper 'Some implicit common factors in diverse methods of psychotherapy: At last the Dodo said, "Everybody has won and all must have prizes"'(Rosenzweig, 1936). This paper foreshadows the development of a 'common-factors' approach to therapy (to be discussed further in Chapter 11) in the second half of the 20th century. The common factors perspective and agenda is crucial to understanding the development of pluralism and its potential importance, since it challenges the basis of so much research. Most therapy research taken seriously by policymakers and providers assumes that effectiveness as a variable is determined by approach. If this assumption is erroneous, then so are the results. The implications of Rosenzweig's paper have led to practitioners and researchers talking with each other about the 'dodo bird verdict' (e.g. Cooper, 2008; Wampold & Imel, 2015), with some advocating for this verdict to be accepted and others challenging it (see also Purton, 2016).

In the 1940s, psychotherapy 'was the province of medicine' (Wampold & Imel, 2015, p. 20), so Rogers, a psychologist and not a doctor, was not allowed to use the title 'psychotherapist'. Although there were no regulations to prevent non-medical practitioners from using the title in the UK, psychotherapy was, in effect, seen as a medical practice until the end of the 1960s (e.g., see Balfour, 1995). So, borrowing the title 'counsellor', which had previously been associated with careers guidance and education, to enable practice by non-medical practitioners might be seen as a completely pragmatic move intended to enable non-medical practitioners to practise; however, this division of practitioners into 'counsellors' and 'psychotherapists' has become another unresolved area of dispute and controversy in the field. Some practitioners support this distinction (e.g. McLeod, 2013), and others do not (e.g. BACP, 2010). Although 'psychotherapy' could eventually be practised by non-medical practitioners, the wish to hold on to a perceived difference and/or superiority continued, adding another dimension to the steady increase of divisions within the practice of therapy. This development in the profession illustrates conflicts that continued to manifest around medicine/science/expert models of therapy versus philosophy/art/facilitator models, with the latter being more associated with humanistic therapies.

Rosenthal and Frank (1956) 'recommended the use of placebo-type controls in psychotherapy research to establish the specificity as well as efficacy of psychotherapy' (Wampold & Imel, 2015, p. 24). This kind of research laid the basis for 'conceptualizing psychotherapy as a medical treatment' (2015, p. 24) – a conceptualisation that is still with us and has become a point of division between practitioners, who either support or deny the practice of therapy as a medical endeavour.

Nevertheless, therapists within medical systems are in competition with other psychological professionals, and in order to survive and thrive within those systems, they need to prove equivalence, if not superiority, to those other professionals; hence the willingness of therapists and their representatives to conform to medical models and their associated research methodologies. In particular, psychiatrists who, on the whole, pushed a biological model with treatments based on medications practised in a way that enabled 'numerous double-blind placebo trials' (Task Force on Promotion and Dissemination of Psychological Procedures, 1995). If therapists wanted to compete with psychiatrists, they needed to allow therapy to be conceptualised as something much akin to a medication and not to compete on the level of actual efficacy but on the level of being able to adhere to privileged research methodologies. In order to do this and establish 'empirically supported treatments' (ESTs), all that needed to happen was for therapy to accept and 'adopt a Medical Model' (Wampold & Imel, 2015, p. 27). In the medical model, a 'biological explanation' is usually the basis for explaining a 'disease or illness', so the 'only modification needed for the psychotherapy version [was] that the biological explanation [be] transformed into a psychological explanation' (2015, p. 28). The survival of therapists within medical systems gradually intensified the relationship of therapy with the medical model. This politicised a fundamental divide within therapy between those supportive of the medical model and those uncomfortable with its gradually increasing dominance over the conceptualisation and practice of therapy. It might be argued that this trend reflected an internal split within the therapeutic profession itself, but it can also be seen as a pragmatic position taken by a professional group in order to have the opportunity to have dialogue and gain acceptance with the medical establishment within which they hoped to practise.

The medical model insists on the idea of 'treatments' that have an effect beyond 'placebo', and many therapy researchers comply with this imposition of a medical model on what is, arguably, not a treatment but a dialogue based on rhetoric (e.g. Szasz, 1988). Research into therapy process has actually decreased, probably because although more useful for therapists and clients the culture of ESTs has no need for it (e.g. Wampold & Imel, 2015). Therapists and the bodies that represent them need to push for non-medicalised ways of researching therapy, to reflect more accurately the views and experiences of clients and therapists. Additionally, it is important that the tendency of a 'medical model – RCT – new public management' complex to reduce the diversity of practice (i.e. a monistic rather than a pluralistic model of provision, especially concerning therapy in healthcare systems) is challenged (e.g. Boe et al., 2024). In the meantime, the therapy wars continue.

Therapy Wars

I hypothesise that divisive debates about therapy, which I characterise as 'therapy wars', following Saltzman and Norcross (1990), are fuelled by the themes of Chapters 5 to 7, namely contentious issues about 1) therapeutic approaches and identities, 2) how flexible or rigid the practice of therapy should be and 3) the importance (or not) of the relationship, with all three of these contentious issues related to fundamental divisions between therapists based on scientific/medical versus artistic/relational attitudes towards the practice of therapy, as discussed in the previous section.

It is also my hypothesis that these divisive debates have led to the evolution of three major trends in therapy which, implicitly, attempt to resolve the divisiveness of these issues: firstly, the practice of metacommunication (a significant feature of pluralistic therapy), in which dialogue between therapists and clients can determine how therapy is practised (rather than relying on off-the-shelf, one-size-fits-all applications of whatever brand of therapy is currently deemed to be best by those outside the actual therapeutic relationship); secondly, the postmodern/pluralistic perspective, which acknowledges that increasing our understandings of what works in therapy is a worthy endeavour but is destined to be 'ever not quite' (Araujo & Osbeck, 2023) and, therefore, the uncertainty that exists in therapy – from the phenomenological and microcosmic experience of the therapeutic dyad across to nomothetic and idiographic research and abstract theorising – must not only be tolerated but accepted, and even celebrated (e.g. Loewenthal, 2011); thirdly, a drive towards theorising how to practise therapy based on 'common factors', a popular aspect of the integrative therapy movement. These trends will be discussed in further detail in Chapters 9 to 11.

Therapy Wars and Pluralistic Therapy

The pluralistic therapy agenda, in my view, and at least implicitly, is a 'peace' agenda for the psychological therapy professions, which also relates to issues and debates about professionalisation and regulation (explored in a later section). Therefore, how therapists support or challenge its tenets and practices is important in contributing to understanding the ongoing struggle of the therapy profession with embracing difference and presenting itself as a united front for its survival and progress. It is worth analysing how the pluralistic agenda is both failing and succeeding to convince therapists that it is important or useful.

If a pluralistic agenda takes hold, there will be significant implications for how commissioning bodies, therapists, trainers, and researchers develop and focus their practices. For instance, accepting a pluralistic view of therapy has profound implications for professional identity (Hemsley, 2013).

I see the publication of *Pluralistic Counselling and Psychotherapy* (Cooper & McLeod, 2011) as a significant 'critical juncture' (e.g. Aldridge, 2011) when the conceptualisation of 'pluralistic therapy' became widespread within the profession and ignited debates about the idea of pluralistic therapy in itself and, also, other related issues.

One major issue is the compatibilities and incompatibilities of modern versus postmodern paradigms in relation to pluralistic therapy. This is central to understanding the debates around pluralistic therapy and related issues and will be explored further in Chapter 10. The subtleties and complexities of modernism and postmodernism deserve more space than can be adequately addressed in this chapter, but for now, it is enough to acknowledge the importance of postmodernism versus modernism concerning multiple conflicts in the therapy world.

Similarly, it could be argued that there is a fundamental conceptual split between symptom-focussed therapies (such as CBT), what Halmos (1965) called 'mechanotherapy', which is aimed at perceived illnesses within a whole person, and holistic/narrative therapies, which are aimed at the entire person and whose 'illnesses' might improve from exploration of the whole self (e.g. Grogan, 2013). This split, which is one reflection of the culture/counter-culture discourses from the 1960s and 1970s onwards, forms part of the current debates about pluralism. Pluralistic therapy argues for the provision of humanistic therapies, whether by individual practitioners or mental health services. Humanistic therapies usually have an ethic of working with people over symptoms, and, in that sense, the pluralistic agenda is a way of getting humanistic therapies back into circulation. In this way, pluralistic therapy might be seen to be as much about rescuing humanistic therapies from their falling out of favour with established providers as offering choice and its other ideals – a brazen attempt to challenge the dominance of symptom-based therapies with a more holistic approach.

The push for pluralistic approaches to therapy by Cooper and McLeod has fostered and continues to foster controversy. One of the more noticeable discussions took place in the pages of *Therapy Today* magazine, in which pluralistic therapy was featured as a 'debate', with Michael Owens arguing 'against factionalism' (Owens, 2014) and Chris Molyneux arguing for a recognition of 'the problem with pluralism' (Molyneux, 2014). The latter piece criticised the approach of the eighth of Cooper and McLeod's (2011) frequently asked questions: viz. you cannot mix up different philosophical and psychological assumptions. Molyneux specifically argues that the PCA cannot be mixed with other approaches, such as CBT, if the PCA is deeply and philosophically understood. This understanding of the PCA as incompatible with other approaches (if the therapist strays into practising in ways that impede the client's sense of being 'self-directing' and the 'expert' of their own life) is quite widespread amongst its practitioners and theoreticians (e.g. see Mearns et al., 2013, p. 201). The Owens/Molyneux articles set off another flurry of letters arguing for and against both purism and pluralism. It is a perennial topic of debate that now refers to pluralism as an identifying label distinct from integrationism and eclecticism.

More recently, also in *Therapy Today*, while promoting a new edition of *The Tribes of the Person-Centred Nation* (*TTOTPCN*) (2024a), Cooper, McLeod, and others made arguments that while respect for the original conceptualisations of Rogers's PCA is deserved there is also a danger that the PCA becomes stuck in its past and unresponsive to research (see Jackson, 2024). The issue of whether the core conditions of unconditional positive regard, empathy, and congruence are 'sufficient' – which should be a debate familiar to most students and practitioners of humanistic therapy – has become a point of contention between pluralists and purists (even if they do not use those terms to describe themselves). Cooper and others suggest that often the conditions are not sufficient or, at least, they are not sufficient for all clients all of the time. Conversely, other practitioners believe that they absolutely are sufficient when skilfully practised. In the latest edition of *TTOTPCN*, 'pluralistic person-centred therapy' has its own chapter: for some PCA practitioners, this might be viewed as a contradiction in terms, possibly an affront. For Cooper's pluralistic take on the PCA, collaboration, metacommunication, and shared decision-making are the practices that can be brought into the therapeutic relationship, which take it out of only adhering to the core conditions while still remaining person-centred at heart. This is a view not shared by all.

Some people characterise this challenge to the purism of the PCA as a challenge to dogmatic thinking. Andrew Reeves references Rogers (1961) himself as suggesting that knowledge/research will 'bring about the gradual demise of "schools" of psychotherapy', and that 'there will be less and less emphasis upon dogmatic and purely theoretical formulations' (Rogers cited in Jackson, 2024, p. 23). This is suggestive of a more integrative, generic form of therapy and an implicit assumption that the demise of schools of therapy is necessarily a good thing. From a pluralistic perspective, the existence of different, even contradictory and irreconcilable philosophies and practices of therapy, while challenging, is something to be tolerated and not wished away. This is an instance of the often muddled theoretical grappling with integrative versus pluralistic attitudes to therapy. It is still unclear to me, after immersing myself in these debates for many years now, whether those who advocate for pluralistic therapy are actually more enamoured of the idea of a generic therapy rather than celebrating the diversity of the therapies we already have and which will continue to come into being as therapy evolves.

Ani de la Prida (2020), as a person-centred practitioner and now an advocate of the pluralistic approach, insists that it is possible to be both person-centred and pluralistic. She says that she agrees that the core conditions are sufficient, but that descriptor 'feels to me a little dry … we can survive on bread and water, it is sufficient. But … maybe a little jam or marmite would be nice?' (2020).

Therapy Wars and Regulation: Statutory and Otherwise

The importance of regulation, particularly SR, is a significant controversy in the background of debates about pluralism. The most recent attempt to statutorily regulate psychological therapies in the UK failed. One of many reasons for this is a consequence of the pluralism of approaches, ideologies, and professional titles within the field. From a regulatory point of view, the pluralism of psychological therapies is an inconvenience, since regulation requires clarity, and for the psychological therapies, with so many opposing and confusing positions, that clarity does not exist.

It is difficult to foresee what SR would actually mean for therapists – to assert what would or would not happen – but one possibility might be the demarcation of approaches/practices, leading to professional inflexibility across approaches and professions (Morgan-Ayrs, 2016). In this sense, the issue of regulation hovers in the background of debates about pluralism and purism because how the professions might be regulated has implications for how pluralistic perspectives and practices might thrive – or not – in such regulatory frameworks. This is especially true for the public sector, if less so for private practice. Morgan-Ayrs (2016) has concerns that regulation could lead to 'the session being a tick box series of tasks to be covered in such and such a way' (p. 11), which seems similar to how Cooper and McLeod (e.g. 2011) sometimes articulate their version of pluralistic practice. Therefore, it could be argued that their framework is not just tailored for favoured models of research but also for potential regulatory frameworks. This regulation-friendly therapy differs from what Morgan-Ayrs (2016) describes as the 'spontaneous conversation associated with humanistic or most psychoanalytic sessions' (p. 31); however, the intangible nature of therapeutic practice goes against what regulatory bodies want to hear. For instance, Szasz (1988) asserts that therapy is nothing more than, at best, rhetorical conversation and, therefore, cannot logically be seen as a medical treatment. This might be a valid argument, but it is one that challenges the notion of psychological therapies as 'health' treatments and, by implication, the placing of these practices in a 'health' service or 'health' insurance schemes. Indeed, the resistance to the medical model from – in a broad sense – humanistic practitioners leads some to suggest that therapy does not even belong in the NHS (e.g. Lawton & Nash, 2013), since, from a humanistic point of view, mental suffering is not a 'health' issue, but rather a state of mind based in existential conditions common to all of us.

A subtextual message of the intense debates and calls for regulation and professionalisation, often in the name of protecting clients, is that therapists are not professional enough, even dangerous. While it is true, as in any profession, that some practitioners may lack conscientiousness and/or skills, on the whole, the amount of thought and energy which goes into individual practices and the amount of continuous learning practitioners are willing to undertake for the benefit of clients is distinctly impressive. Supervision, case studies, and post-qualification CPD may not produce the evidence required for public sector provision of therapy, but they do provide the best forms of learning for therapists – learning which in turn provides the best therapeutic experiences for clients.

Therapy Wars, Research, and CBT

For non-CBT practitioners, the dominance of CBT in comparison to their own chosen modalities is also of concern. This is a major factor in conflicts about therapeutic approaches: there is a perception that CBT is 'winning' because CBT organisations have seized the power of research to drive commercial interests. However, the acceptance that CBT has indisputably won the research battle is not universal, and much research continues to support a sceptical position regarding its perceived supremacy (e.g. Barkham et al., 2017; Pybis et al., 2017). Some research demonstrates, amongst other things, that 'it's the relationship' (discussed previously) rather than particular approaches which are the most effective 'ingredient' in therapy.

Overall, the privileging of CBT as the 'treatment of choice' (e.g. Royal College of Psychiatrists, 2024) is challenged by many therapists and researchers, who see CBT's claimed efficacy as 'overestimated' (e.g. Riddle, 2024). Dalal (2018) critiques the privileging of CBT as facilitated by neoliberalism and managerialism (for instance, NPM), in which obsessions with perceived efficiency and goals to achieve such efficiency often lead to worse outcomes in many areas, but especially in the provision of therapy. In *Why Not CBT? Against and For CBT Revisited* (Loewenthal & Proctor, 2018), similar themes are discussed comprehensively and give voice to both sides of the debate.

Therapy Wars are OK

Samuels (2011/1997) argues that the various debates in therapy, of which the debate about approaches is just one, are a way to define what therapy *is*. In that sense, 'debate, dispute and difference' (p. 222) are beneficial for therapy. Pluralism, he argues, is not about a woolly tolerance but a hard acceptance of different and emotionally charged positions. He actively wishes to encourage the disputes and arguments associated with the *fact* of pluralism (by which I mean the fact that there are different and sometimes irreconcilable positions about phenomena), which accords with others who advocate pluralism as a philosophical viewpoint which opposes the 'demand for consensus' (e.g. Rescher, 1993). In that sense, these debates are positive for the profession.

Concluding Thoughts

I have named this chapter 'Therapy Wars' because this term encapsulates conflicts within the profession, which are, arguably, one basis for the manifestation of pluralistic therapy as a potential pathway to the resolution of such conflicts. The use of this phrase to describe factionalism within the therapy professions has also been articulated by others (e.g. Burkeman, 2016; Saltzman & Norcross, 1990).

These conflicts are characterised by defensiveness and aggressiveness, often rooted in fear and divisive 'us/them' attitudes. They also reflect a modern (as opposed to postmodern) desire for certainty and discomfort with uncertainty, paralleling a view of therapy as something based on preconceived ideas (as opposed to a creative, exploratory, dialogical, and phenomenological experience of discovery). Therapists who might be insecure about their practice can obtain a sense of security by adhering steadfastly to the tenets of a model.

One implicit difference between therapists who engage more passionately in these conflicts and those who are more cynical and disconnected from them is their different attitudes toward therapeutic theories. There are different degrees of ambivalence towards theories as a basis for practice. Such ambivalence might make it more difficult for some therapists to engage in debates that are often highly theoretical and dominated by voices that assume the importance of coherent theoretical underpinnings for therapeutic practice. For instance, overly enthusiastic embracing of particular theoretical perspectives can be therapeutically counter-productive. Theories can get in the way of the therapeutic relationship whereby the theory may act almost like a filter between therapist and client if the therapist is viewing the client through a theory rather than the phenomenological relationship (see Boe et al., 2024): 'reality risks being hidden behind the veil of knowledge' (p. 2).

Conflicts in the therapy professions, however, do not solely come from such relatively benign causes as fighting for ideological and pragmatic perceptions of what makes therapists and therapy effective and worthwhile; they also come from more mundane and calculated motives which have commercial/professional implications such as to achieve political and economic ascendancy or supremacy. Arguing for institutional validation of some approaches but not others has 'real-world' implications for the success and failure of therapies and therapists. The practice of therapy – especially with so many practitioners operating in the private sector (e.g. BACP, 2017) – is a highly competitive commercial enterprise (e.g. Clark, 2002), and therapists are – even on a casual level – aware of their need to 'sell' their services. Approaches and techniques such as Acceptance and Commitment Therapy (ACT), CBT, MBCT, and Eye Movement Desensitisation and Reprocessing (EMDR) have undeniable commercial value, and sometimes therapists will train in them or gain post-qualification credentials in them for purely financial motives.

The emphasis on differences between approaches and the branding of such approaches can be seen as just a kind of refranchising, repackaging, and rebranding of very similar ideas, with 'common factors' (see Chapter 11 for more on this) doing most of the work despite any particular therapeutic approach with which practitioners identify (e.g. Miller et al., 1997; Saltzman & Norcross, 1990). This notion of rebranding the same ideas under a different name is, of course, also an accusation that can be directed at pluralistic therapy itself (e.g. Ong et al., 2020). The idealistic vision of a more tolerant and open-minded profession, articulated by those sympathetic to conceptions of pluralistic theory and practice, is perceived by some therapists as being just as motivated by commercial and professional concerns.

Cooper and McLeod concede that 'many therapists already think, and practise, in a way that is consistent with the pluralistic approach' (Cooper & McLeod, 2011, p. 157) but insist that theirs is the first comprehensive articulation of how many therapists have been practising. They also perceive their pluralistic practice as 'uniquely inclusive and collaborative' (p. 157). Importantly, they emphasise how their 'framework' enables research to be carried out in ways that previous articulations of this kind of practice have not. Indeed, pluralistic therapy theorists' agenda in promoting the importance of research becomes increasingly apparent as it evolves (e.g. Cooper et al., 2024). The relevance of this to common factors and the future of therapy will be elaborated upon in Chapters 11 and 12, respectively.

Chapter 9

Metacommunication

Metacommunication: Talking about Talking, Collaboration, and Shared Decision-Making

Metacommunication (Cooper & McLeod, 2011), or 'talking about talking', involves open collaborations between therapists and clients that inform how they want to work together, rather than assuming the methods of the practitioner's preferred model are needed and wanted: it is a major feature and concept of the pluralistic framework (e.g. Brown & Smith, 2023). Smith and de la Prida (2021) describe it as 'talking about what is going on; a way of observing therapy, making insights and comments about the process and interactions and inviting open feedback' (p. 111). Metacommunication can facilitate the therapeutic process within one approach, allow movement between approaches with one therapist, or signal that a client might perhaps be better off with another therapist – either because the therapist does not want to work in ways the client wants to or because they do not feel they have the competence or skills to do so. McLeod (2018) characterises its use in pluralistic therapy as a 'general strategy that supports collaboration and shared decision-making' (p. 83).

Metacommunication as a concept is, in some ways, easier to grasp than how it is concretely delivered in actual sessions. Sarah Cantwell (2022), on the basis of transcribed sessions to which she has applied a conversational analysis, suggests a 'conversational manoeuvre' of 'de-specifying', which 'involves providing a structure and guidance to help clients talk about their preferences, but then making sure it is not so rigid or directive that it leads a client down any particular path'. The general point Cantwell makes is that the idea of metacommunication needs skilful application in order for it to be effective. When practitioners argue about the pros and cons of metacommunication, clarity is needed about what they mean by the term in actual practice and in the actual conversations that take place between therapists and clients. Cantwell (2018) suggests that how therapists create, or open, 'opportunity for meta-therapeutic dialogue' (p. 274) can be more or less complex or problematic depending on contextual factors, such as whether it is the right time in the therapeutic process to prioritise a more empathic or more problem-solving mode. Importantly, if questions are used in metacommunication, these must facilitate the

DOI: 10.4324/9781003468332-9

'inviting' of the 'client's own ideas', and Cantwell also warns against 'pursuing answers from clients' (p. 275). From her conversational analysis, there are many recommendations about how metacommunication can be more or less effective at the granular level of actual dialogical interactions between therapists and clients.

McLeod (2018) traces the history of the concept of 'metacommunication' back to the 1950s and family system theorists such as Gregory Bateson. Regarding pluralistic therapy, the use of the term is most relevant in Rennie's (1994) paper on 'clients' deference'. This research paper suggested that clients often defer to the therapist not because they want to but out of politeness, a lack of metacommunication or ineffective metacommunication when it occurs. One implication of the paper is that more effective communication with clients, especially via metacommunication about the therapeutic process, would benefit them. The pluralistic emphasis on collaboration and metacommunication can be seen as a response to the therapeutic problems highlighted in Rennie's paper.

Rennie (1998) identifies four main types of metacommunication:

1 The speaker may disclose to the other person the *intention* behind what the speaker has said or is about to say.
2 The speaker may disclose his or her reactions to what the other person has said (*impact*).
3 The speaker may invite the other to reveal the *intention* behind what the other has said.
4 The speaker may invite the other to disclose his or her reaction to what the speaker has said (*impact*).

(Rennie, 1998, cited in McLeod, 2018, p. 84)

Metacommunication is the most central and distinctive feature of pluralistic therapy. In 2012, Cooper and McLeod also usefully distinguished a particular type of metacommunication within a therapeutic context as 'meta-therapeutic communication' (MTC) (Cooper & McLeod, 2012). Papayianni and Cooper (2017) define MTC thus:

a form of metacommunication which focuses specifically on the way that therapy is, has been or could be done, with the aim of optimising its helpfulness to the individual client. This distinguishes it from other forms of metacommunication, such as working in the "here-and-now" or transference work.

(p. 173)

Cantwell (2018) further suggests that the concept of MTC (also called meta-therapeutic dialogue by her and others):

involves substantial conceptual intersection with several existing therapeutic concepts and approaches, including responsiveness, meta-communication,

collaboration, working alliance, negotiation, therapy personalization and elici-
tation of client preferences, shared decision-making and resource-oriented and
dialogical perspectives.

(p. 59)

In this chapter, I use the term 'metacommunication' as the default, as it encom-
passes more than MTC on its own.

One purpose of metacommunication is to devolve power away from therapists
and towards clients. This is, arguably, good for the therapeutic process in itself
but also, if taken up collectively, could be a path to peace and reconciliation in the
profession more widely. If clients are allowed to decide what kind of therapy they
want and with what kind of therapists, then, at least in theory, the need for therapists and other stakeholders to argue about the efficacy of and place for various
therapies dissolves. 'Why not ask clients what they want and give it to them?' is
the rhetorical question behind the call for metacommunication at the political level.
This open and informative communication about therapeutic choices does not just
occur at the beginning of therapy, for example, in assessment but throughout, so
that clients can choose how therapy can be tailored for them individually, either
with one therapist/therapy or a series of therapists/therapies.

As well as devolving power away from therapists and towards clients, the practice
of metacommunication might also allow for a devolving of power away from the
'expertise' of professional bodies, researchers, and providers to clients themselves
and their own unique, contextual positioning, which often challenges attempts to
categorise and define. In this sense, metacommunication holds promise not just for
empowering clients but also for empowering therapists whose approaches have
not been 'approved' by research: it has the potential to be 'political' as well as
'personal'. In other words, in contexts in which so-called 'evidence-based' therapies marginalise therapies without evidence from privileged methodologies, there
could be a direct challenge from both clients and therapists to demand the therapies
and the therapists that they actually want rather than have their 'choices' dictated
to them by pseudo-scientific bodies such as NICE.

The concept of 'shared decision-making' referred to earlier comes from the
medical field and can be seen as an additional variant of the medical model. In
defining it, Coulter and Collins (2011) say that 'it involves the provision of evidence-based information about options, outcomes and uncertainties' (p. vii). If
therapists and clients are similarly constrained within a narrow evidence base, the
potential for flexibility and open choices will decrease. Ultimately, how metacommunication manifests and decisions are arrived at, if operated within constrain-
ing paradigms, might offer more or less empowerment for therapists and clients,
as limiting choices to 'evidence-based' therapies leaves hardly any choice at all.
Overall, however, shared decision-making via the process of metacommunication
has the potential to move therapy away from paternalistic models of provision in
which therapists hold the power to one where power over the process of therapy is
'shared equally' (Norcross & Cooper, 2021, p. 11).

Norcross and Cooper (2021) support shared decision-making because it is a way of 'personalizing' therapy, which they see as essential because 'individual differences, client heterogeneity, individual variability, our undeniable uniqueness' means that people 'vary widely in how to achieve [relief from suffering]' (2021, p. 11). In some ways, the idea of personalising therapy is a simpler, more direct aim for the therapy field. It holds similar ambitions to pluralistic therapy and integrative therapy (pluralistic therapy's 'cousin', or 'parent', or 'child', or 'ally', depending on one's perspective), and its meaning is less ambiguous than the terms pluralistic or integrative. In addition, it does not infer the need for a framework or approach to surround it. Therefore, the idea of personalising therapy does not fall into the same traps of theoretical and philosophical argumentation that both pluralistic and integrative theorists struggle with: one either agrees or disagrees that therapy needs to become more personalised. Moreover, personalising therapy 'improves success and decreases dropouts' (2021, p. 33). To argue for personalising therapy is not to argue for a newer or better approach/framework but more for how we can personalise therapy with what we already have and might have in the future.

Pluralistic therapy theorists seem unsure of how therapists should use evidence to influence their collaborative choices with clients. For instance, Cooper et al. (2016) assert that 'therapists should familiarise themselves with the evidence on what works in therapy: both at the intervention level and the level of different methods' (p. 50). Yet in a different chapter in the same book, McLeod and Sundet (2016) characterise pluralistic therapy 'as a form of radical eclecticism' (p. 160), which 'means ... to pick and choose without these choices being dictated or constrained by demands for logical and theoretical coherence' (p. 161). The latter approach is bounded by working with the clients' preferences, but it nevertheless seems to have less of an emphasis on evidence gained outside of actually working with a particular client. The 'evidence' is only gathered from particular experiences of particular clients from particular sessions, a so-called 'client-directed outcome-informed' therapy (e.g. Duncan & Miller, 2000). This approach to evidence and practice is more pluralistic in spirit, as it values the particular to inform the whole rather than accepting that generalised evidence is necessarily of use to any particular individual.

Some therapists are less convinced and more cynical about the importance of metacommunication to and for clients. The establishment of trust between therapists and clients is seen as more important. In other words, there can be an assumption that clients do not want to discuss the technicalities of how therapy may or may not proceed. Clients want support and might prefer to just get on with talking rather than talking about talking. In a pluralistic spirit, Cooper and McLeod concede that sometimes clients want therapists to take the lead and acknowledge that metacommunication is unsuitable for these kinds of clients for part or all of the therapeutic process. Cooper and McLeod suggest being sensitive to these kinds of clients and 'adjusting accordingly' (Cooper & McLeod, 2011, p. 155).

The evidence base for the value of metacommunication is inconclusive. Some research suggests that the impact on outcomes is small (e.g. Duncan et al., 2010), while other research suggests that clients value it and especially value receiving their 'preferred intervention' (Cooper et al., 2016, p. 45; Swift et al., 2011, p. 307).

One of the main ways in which pluralistic therapy aims to transcend 'school-ism' and, in my interpretation, offers a 'diplomatic attempt at resolution' to the conflicts between therapeutic approaches is via the practice of MTC: MTC forms one foundation of its attempt to practise 'collaborative integration' (Cooper & Dryden, 2016).

The perceived need for MTC depends on various factors, one of which is where practitioners position themselves on the flexibility–rigidity continuum (see Chapter 6): the more flexible a practitioner, the more approaches and techniques that practitioner might use, and therefore, arguably, the more there is a need for MTC and collaboration. In turn, how comfortable therapists and clients are with flexibility and MTC depends on their relationship to, and tolerance of, uncertainty and understanding. Differences of opinion about how flexible therapists should be is one aspect that appears in the debates about pluralism; respect for uncertainty, as well as understanding, might be seen as one 'diplomatic attempt' to resolve this is-sue. I term this the 'uncertainty–understanding continuum', to be explored in more detail in the next chapter.

The main challenge of MTC for pluralistic therapy, however, is whether clients might be trusted enough and empowered enough to make up their own minds about what kind of therapist and therapeutic approach they want. In the NHS, and more broadly in medical model thinking applied to the practice and provision of therapy, the current assumption is that expert researchers need to evaluate different thera-pies for the benefit of clients with particular symptoms. Perhaps it might be easier, cheaper, and more effective to ask clients of sufficient capacity and knowledge what they would prefer. This is an idea that, as far as I am aware, has not been proposed, let alone entertained, despite the patient-centred rhetoric of the NHS.

There is also the danger that the concept of MTC mirrors 'contemporary politi-cal drives to privatize healthcare and conceptually individualize the social, political and economic causes of psychological distress' (Cantwell, 2018).

Metacommunication and Goals

Cooper and McLeod (2007) are fond of being explicit and clear with clients about therapeutic goals. In terms of metacommunication, they write, 'Another important skill … involves checking out with the client that the work is on track to fulfil a previously-agreed goal' (Cooper & McLeod, 2007, p. 137). So, a therapist who dis-agrees with the implicit value of metacommunication (Cooper & McLeod, 2007; Kiesler, 1988) or goal-setting of any kind would not be seen in their envisaged plu-ralistic protocol as practising effectively. Cooper and McLeod argue that their use of the word 'goals' is meant quite loosely as 'goals that are *already there*, in terms of being implicit in the structure of the person's engagement with his or her life-space' (2007, italics in original). However, some practitioners, such as Rowan, are uncomfortable with the concept of goals: 'goals get in the way of the relationship and distort it mightily' (Rowan, 2015). For other practitioners, it might be that this word/domain and its relation to the associated explanation of a possible pluralistic practice is merely misunderstood or misconstrued. Nevertheless, misunderstood or not, the terminology of their model might be one reason for a more general resistance by some parts of the therapy profession to engage with the model for pluralistic practice.

Brown and Smith (2023) assert that 'therapeutic goals are essential to pluralistic therapy' (p. 71), and this idea has become more firmly embedded in the pluralistic therapy field. Such a 'rule' could be seen as anti-pluralistic in that it does not, at first glance, include therapists such as Rowan, who might prioritise working with the therapeutic process in the present, with any future ambitions for therapy outcomes only implicit. One of the main critiques of pluralistic therapy is that it reflects an 'anything goes' attitude – perhaps the emphasis on goals acts as a defence against such accusations. With the setting of goals and the other two pragmatic concepts of tasks and methods, what I characterise as a 'Holy Trinity', foundational to the protocols of pluralistic therapy as a named practice, pluralistic therapy theorists can more easily claim a logical and coherent basis for it. Underlying such concerns, however, are 'modern' values in thrall to wanting to demonstrate coherence and logic versus a 'postmodern' acceptance of incoherence and irrationality. This modern/postmodern split within the therapy profession will be explored further in the next chapter.

Brown and Smith (2023) do acknowledge that setting goals 'can be seen as too restrictive, with an emphasis on change and "doing" rather than accepting and "being"'(p. 75) but overall emphasise the evidence which supports the value of goal setting (pp. 73–74). Further to embracing goal-setting, they also align themselves with monitoring the progress towards these goals via deliberate 'metacommunication and feedback' (p. 92). This might occur in dialogue, but they also promote the use of forms. Proponents of pluralistic therapy are often openly fond of forms to monitor and measure, and, again, this causes some divisions of opinion within the therapy profession.

Cooper, in more recent years, with the publication of *Integrating Counselling and Psychotherapy* (2019a), has responded to the criticisms around goals by revising what he means in relation to them as a more holistic, rather than mechanistic, conception of 'directionality', which he defines as a 'forward-moving, active quality of human being' (2019a, p. 6). Importantly, he offers a more comprehensive analysis of the multiple dimensions of goals within this broader directionality, which makes a complete dismissal of them (as made by Rowan) more difficult to justify and is demanding of more complex critiques.

Chapter 10

Uncertainty, Understanding, Modernism, and Postmodernism

Uncertainty and Understanding

A significant issue facing therapy for all those involved (clients, therapists, re-searchers, providers) is navigating the need to understand, when uncertainty so often prevails. Therapists searching for feelings of certainty about their practice can easily be tempted to stick to narrow bases of understanding in terms of approach and techniques. If strict boundaries are put in place about what belongs to a particular approach, and/or if the rightness of that approach is substantially accepted, then it is reassuring for therapists (especially those more inexperienced) to feel confident that how they are conducting therapy is correct, safe, and less susceptible to complaint (formally or informally).

In contrast, many practitioners support the idea that therapeutic practice needs to accept 'ambiguity, not knowing, the intuitive and the mysterious' (House, 2016, p. 149). Nevertheless, the 'literature suggests that trainees have a need for certainty in the early stages of a career in order to reduce anxiety as the therapist moves from training towards professional individuation and expertise' (Thompson & Cooper, 2012, p. 65). Thompson and Cooper further add that by following a pluralistic approach 'there is less certainty about the way that one should work with a client; instead there must be an acceptance of the underlying philosophical values of pluralism and a commitment to working without certainty' (p. 65).

I propose that there is an *uncertainty–understanding continuum* that exists in and between clients and therapists. Therapists have varying degrees of professional uncertainty about their practice in particular and about therapy in general. Feelings of uncertainty are, perhaps, most likely to be experienced before or during training, when a sense of what being a therapist entails is at its most elusive. For instance, when I enrolled for my humanistic training, I had little idea who Carl Rogers was, even though person-centred therapy was a central influence on the course structure. When one knows little about therapy, staying close to a particular model can allay fears around practice; nevertheless, uncertainty can manifest in various ways, even when therapists are relatively experienced.

After training, uncertainty persists about what to do or how to be a therapist. Qualifications and practical experience gained on placements are, to some extent,

DOI: 10.4324/9781003468332-10

reassuring. Yet, there is still always the unknown of forever new therapeutic encounters (Bott & Howard, 2012) for which therapists can never be absolutely and fully prepared, no matter how great their theoretical or technical know-how. Furthermore, similarly for clients – despite therapist qualifications (and labels such as 'CBT' or 'psychodynamic'), which might offer initial reassurance – in the end, therapy is a human meeting which may or may not facilitate the development of trust (a kind of certainty) and a functional therapeutic relationship.

From a client's perspective, the uncertainty and 'not knowing' that they often bring to a therapeutic encounter forms the basis on which critics of pluralistic therapy question its emphasis on choice, collaboration, and metacommunication (as discussed in the previous chapter). Sometimes, clients do not know what they want from therapy and have little idea of what therapy is or how they might use it. They are just glad to have a therapist and think that therapy will be helpful. Of course, some clients are relatively well-informed and might have experience of different therapies and different therapists or have done other kinds of therapeutic work for their own personal healing and development. These clients often know about different approaches and how they may or may not fit their needs. Clients can also be highly emotionally aware and literate and have more certainty about how and with whom they want to work; collaborating on *how* to proceed with this type of client is arguably less problematic.

In Cooper and McLeod's pluralistic therapy, their tolerance of uncertainty seems to be diluted with an undue emphasis on suggested protocols and the encouragement of routine monitoring of sessions by therapists. It is almost as if the very uncertainty, which from a pluralistic perspective is welcome, is only acceptable if therapists and clients keep a keen eye on it, as if it is in some way inherently dangerous.

Cooper and his colleagues are also heavily invested in proving the efficacy of therapeutic processes and outcomes. This goes against sentiments such as Samuels's, which 'proposes the psychotherapist as the archetypal trickster, who has no coherent psychological project, but may end up doing good by accident' (Proctor, 2016). From a pluralistic perspective, this is a view worthy of consideration but quite far from the paradigm of research and practice that Cooper's pluralistic therapy encourages. The spirit of pragmatism and rationalism – there is little doubt of his good intentions in ensuring the provision of therapy for as many people as possible – prevails over tolerating therapy as a social construction riddled with uncertainties and unpredictability.

The tolerance of uncertainty in psychodynamic therapy has been compared to John Keats's '"negative capability", the capacity to be "in Mysteries, uncertainties and doubts, without any irritable reaching after facts and reason"'(Spurling, 2016, p. 126). Spurling suggests that trying 'to understand what [is] happening in therapy' (p. 126) stops therapists from listening to their clients: thinking about 'ideas' in a session can mean that therapists are not listening as closely to their clients as they might be. The importance of embracing uncertainty from a psychodynamic point of view is emphasised by Spurling (2016), referencing Bion (1970): '[t]he capacity to forget, the ability to eschew desire and understanding, must be regarded as essential discipline for the psycho-analyst' (pp. 51–52). This can justify a rationale for non-directivity, for allowing clients space and privileging their awareness rather than attempting to impose feelings of knowing and certainty. Conscious uncertainty on the part of the therapist, or as a basis for a theoretical approach, implies privileging the client as knowing more about themselves than the therapist. This parallels pluralistic acceptance of uncertainty in therapeutic practice.

Many therapists accept uncertainty as a fundamental part of therapy. But this is not reflected in how therapy is conceived of by providers such as the NHS, who subscribe to an 'audit-driven, calculation-obsessed worldview' (House, 2016, p. 149). House states that

> one of the first casualties of this ideology will be any approach to therapy that sees as central the embracing of ambiguity and dialectical thinking in its practice, and which does not conform to any linear, predictable and controllable process or monolithic logic.
>
> (p. 149)

Similarly, regarding influential research (in terms of research that informs policies), therapists often make sense of practice in ways outside its logical, quantifiable, scientistic, and rational boundaries. This reflects just one aspect of what is sometimes referred to as the 'practice-research gap' (e.g. DeAngelis, 2010). If, as previously mentioned, a therapist's development is one of individuation (e.g. Thompson & Cooper, 2012), then one could expect that as therapists become more experienced they also become less standardised. Therefore, the standardisation of therapy within services becomes a constraint that inhibits how therapists can practise and how therapy can be provided for clients. This is powered by an agenda that has permeated the culture – one seeking to monitor and predict certainty about professional practice, a particularly problematic agenda when applied to therapy.

From a feminist standpoint, the need for certainty can be criticised as part of a 'phallogocentric' culture which is attached to the ideal that it can neatly categorise symptoms, treatments, and outcomes and that everyone is completely sure that they know exactly what they are doing (e.g. Spinelli, 1996). Rizq (2016) criticises this attitude as exemplifying the fear of the messier, disordered aspects of caring in more 'feminine' ways.

Similarly, therapy research can also be critiqued as reflecting the phallogocentric culture it is surrounded by in its relentless ambitions towards obtaining certainty about therapeutic processes and outcomes. Additionally, in Goffmanian terms (e.g., see Scott, 2015), one could say that the therapy professions and the research projects behind them are endeavouring to create a good performance for allied professionals and providers so that the profession can survive. Therefore, focusing on the aspects of therapy which are intangible and uncertain – and therapist feelings of not being able to explain and not really know – is a hidden or shadow side of practice shunned by researchers, who purposefully grasp for certainty. There has been some research about uncertainty; for example, Leite and Kuiper (2008) suggest, amongst other things, that 'uncertainty pervades the entire psychotherapeutic process' (p. 55), but overall, it is an under-researched and under-theorised area. Some practitioners (e.g. Yalom, 2015) argue that a different therapy must be provided for each and every client. If that is the case, nothing can be certain about how to practise. This kind of thinking, while popular amongst many practitioners, challenges the very foundation of research, which assumes that best practice can be predicted by what has come before. Critics might counter that these therapists and the problems they pose to research methodologies, accepted fairly easily by other health professionals, perhaps demonstrate a profession not willing and able to come up to the standards imposed on others. However, a profession based on two human beings encountering one another, which is simultaneously a special and an ordinary phenomenon, cannot be as easily analysed as other professions regarding what impedes or facilitates its effectiveness. In my view, therapists, clients, and providers need to be able to tolerate uncertainty as well as reach out for understanding when it comes to allowing the therapeutic encounter (Bott & Howard, 2012) to take its most creative, innovative, and potentially most helpful course.

Modernism and Postmodernism

The everyday terms 'uncertainty' and 'understanding' I have been using thus far can be viewed more philosophically as mirroring differences between modern and postmodern sensibilities. I would argue that therapists often practise from a postmodern perspective, whether they would articulate it as that or not. Postmodern assumptions are 'ground' (in a Gestalt sense) and not necessarily articulated or understood as such. The postmodern perspective is sympathetic to uncertainty and finds itself at odds with cultures insisting on certainty and rigidity. Pluralistic therapy is explicitly postmodern, and pluralism is itself sometimes viewed as synonymous with postmodernism (e.g. Wilber, 2000). The modern cultures within which practitioners with postmodern sensibilities often practise inevitably leads to conflicts, confusions, struggles for empowerment, and feelings of vulnerability and devaluation.

For instance, perhaps the dominance of CBT and the marginalisation of psychodynamic, humanistic and other therapies within bodies such as the NHS reflects a split between modern ways of conceptualising truth and 'best practice' versus postmodern views of uncertainty and practice as contextual rather than generalisable and universal. This modern/postmodern divide is central to difficulties within the profession. In the future, maybe proponents of these two different worldviews can have conversations with each other so that trainers, practitioners, and providers can begin to gain mutual understandings. There might be a way that the deep differences between modern and postmodern worldviews can be reconciled to enable postmodern therapies and therapists to survive in modern healthcare systems. If that cannot happen, then it would seem that there will be no alternative other than for these kinds of practitioners to accept that they will not, and cannot, be understood and so must retreat to private practice, where only economically privileged clients can seek the benefits of such understandings of the therapeutic process.

Polkinghorne (1992) suggested that psychology might be seen as divided into two main camps of 'academic' and 'practice', terming the latter the 'second psychology' (Polkinghorne, 1992, p. 146). The underpinnings of this second psychology are postmodern, in the sense that there are no 'truths' of practice as such, only 'pragmatic usefulness in accomplishing a task' (1992, p. 147) based on the 'actual interactions between practitioners and clients' (p. 146). This interpretation of postmodernism emphasises a 'neopragmatic' (e.g. Rorty, 1991) rather than an ideological or theoretical foundation for practice and sets a tone that supports both proponents of integration and, later, pluralism (e.g. Safran & Messer, 1997; Cooper & McLeod, 2011).

However, House (2011), in response to Cooper and McLeod's launch of pluralistic therapy, in a letter to *Therapy Today*, was sceptical that their pluralistic approach, despite allying itself with postmodernism, engages with postmodern thinking and accused them of being more 'modern' in their 'privileging of "goals", "skills", [and] "methods"'. Some theorists with stronger postmodern leanings question whether therapy has *any* foundations (such as theories) (e.g. Loewenthal, 2011) and, like Polkinghorne, suggest that therapy is better seen as a practice (Loewenthal, 2012, p. 2).

Modern and postmodern conceptualisations of reality and truth are, perhaps, irreconcilable. The modern positivistic paradigm for determining the 'truth' about therapy practice has led to the wholesale ditching of therapies that have not (yet) proven their worth within that paradigm. The motivation for practitioners with more postmodern sensibilities (whether they recognise them as such or not) to prove themselves within that paradigm may or may not be forthcoming.

Pluralism, Postmodernism, and the Person-Centred Approach (PCA)

In more recent years, Cooper, McLeod and others have claimed that their pluralistic therapy, despite its 'goal-directed focus', is part of the 'person-centred tree' (Jackson, 2024, p. 22). Indeed, there is a degree in 'advanced person-centred and pluralistic counselling' at the well-respected Metanoia Institute in London, and one of the principal founders of that degree has written a chapter titled 'pluralistic person-centred therapy' for the latest third edition of *The Tribes of the Person-Centred Nation* (Blunden in Cooper, 2024a). There are some commonalities between the PCA and pluralistic therapy such as valuing 'the inherent capacity of persons to flourish, and draw on their inner knowing as experts on their own experience' (Metanoia, 2024); however, some PCA practitioners are uncomfortable at what they perceive as an 'unnecessary and incompatible' (Ong et al., 2020) encroachment, and a challenge to what they consider to be foundational aspects of the PCA by pluralistic theorists.

One belief perceived by some PCA critics to be foundational to the approach and treated like a *sine qua non* is the belief in the 'actualising tendency'. This belief, framed as fundamental to person-centred philosophy, is perceived as 'radical and political' because the application of it in therapy 'drives the individual to direct their own growth and development' and 'anything other than this subverts the therapeutic process and places power firmly with the "expert" therapist' (Wilson, 2024, p. 13). Avoiding 'expertise' and the perceived power that goes with that expertise in the therapeutic relationship is, for some PCA practitioners, an ultimate value which cannot be transcended by other competing values. For instance, although withholding therapist opinions, psychoeducational interventions, and maybe even questions might facilitate the client's agency, it might be argued that happens at the expense of the therapist's agency. In other words, strict adherence to the therapist not bringing their therapeutic and other related kinds of expertise into the relationship could reduce the dialogical potential of the therapeutic encounter. Perhaps two experts are better than one: the therapist can be an expert as well as the client. Boe et al. (2024) suggest that we 'hold theories at bay (*including our own speculative ontology*) (my italics)' (p. 3). And belief in the actualising tendency can only be framed as both a speculative and ontological position.

The desire of PCA practitioners to distance themselves from the expert position is a valid one and, perhaps, a necessary counterpoint to other approaches (such as CBT) or practices (such as clinical psychology), which can often easily be accused of objectifying and medicalising people when what is needed is a deeper subjective meeting rather than supposedly objective analyses, methodologies, and categorisations. It is more questionable, however, as to whether a foundational belief, such as a belief in the actualising tendency, is truly fundamental for personal healing and growth.

Complicating the issue further is whether foundational beliefs – whether they are of an actualising tendency, or the supposition that the practice of therapy needs to have evidence or research bases, or have materialist or behaviourist assumptions and so forth – are actually of any pragmatic worth in the therapy field *at all* (e.g. Iwakabe, 2003). Boe et al. (2024) suggest that these ontological and epistemological positions, whether credible or not, can get in the way of the 'reality' of clients and therapists in therapeutic encounters. They suggest 'reality is lost' in 'three different frameworks for practice' (2024, p. 5). Firstly, the model-centred framework (such as CBT) reduces the 'reality of the subject' because the people in front of us are 'viewed as an instance of a general problem understood through a theoretical framework' as 'carriers of general phenomena as defined by the model, rather than as real subjects leading real, unique lives' (2024, p. 5). Secondly, the person-centred framework (such as the PCA) is critiqued as being 'monologic in the sense that it is only the logic of the person and their worldview that is made decisive for practice' (2024, p. 6). Both model-centred and person-centred frameworks are characterised by Boe et al. as belonging to the modernist paradigm:

> The model-centred approach is modern in that it is logocentric – based on knowledge, instrumental rationality, and a belief in a continuous enlightenment process with science at its frontiers. The person-centred approach is modern in that it takes the person and an egocentric perspective to be pivotal ("cogito ergo sum"). The ego's actions, experiences, and interpretations are the primary starting point.
>
> (2024, p. 6)

Thirdly, they also conclude that the social constructionist framework (and some other postmodern epistemologies, but not all), despite its potential for overcoming the problems of modernist assumptions, also loses touch with reality 'in the coproduction of representations' because '[r]eality in its own right, prior to being perceived through the lenses of meaning, is lost from sight' (2024, p. 7). Ultimately, Boe et al. conclude that a return to the real is possible by embracing the works of phenomenologists such as Levinas (1985) because he and other phenomenologists 'are not concerned with what the world and another human *are* (ontology/third-person perspective) but what the world, or another human being, *does* with us or *asks of us* as subjects (ethics/first-person perspective)' (2024, p. 7). This serves a dual purpose of 1) avoiding the '[speculations of] [o]ntology and epistemology' (2024, p. 8) and 2) returning to reality (read real encounters between real unique beings) based on phenomenology and ethics. Indeed, Cooper, in response to critiques of pluralistic therapy not having convincing ontological foundations, argues that for him the therapeutic encounter, whether in the PCA or other approaches, needs to privilege the ethical over the ontological (e.g. Cooper, 2024b). Cooper is similarly influenced, like Boe et al., by the phenomenology of Levinas.

So, if from postmodern perspectives which align with a more phenomenological understanding of human experience there can follow scepticism towards the need for paradigms at all, then it also unsurprisingly follows that accusations are made that such lack of any foundational paradigms is anti-scientific, relativistic, and nihilistic (e.g. Woods, 2009).

These characterisations of postmodernism have also come to be used against pluralistic therapy – perceived as and condemned for centring its ideas and framework in postmodernism – especially by some within the PCA (e.g. Ellingham, 2023). Despite Rogers's disillusionment with psychology as an *objective* science, he did want psychology and psychotherapy to be seen as scientific endeavours – only with the subjective aspects more included (e.g. Rogers, 1961). In that sense, a 'Rogerian' attitude to the evolution of therapy might imply that there does need to be a paradigm within which therapy sits and, perhaps implicitly, an ambition that we are working towards a unified field of therapy. This raises a challenge to those who disagree that there needs to be an overarching paradigm for therapy or that the field needs to be unified, or, indeed, that therapy needs to be understood as a science if it is possible to conceive of therapy practice as more akin to an art or craft.

Many in the therapy field support both the desire for scientific credibility and a unifying direction for therapy (even if movement is slow and frustrating). The common factors movement, within the integrative movement more generally, is one potential solution to the problem of the fragmented or diverse nature of therapy. However, from a strong pluralist perspective, the drives towards wanting a unified and scientific paradigm for therapy and, maybe, an idealised future of therapy being an integrated practice of 'evidence-based' common factors is an anathema. From a strong pluralistic perspective, the assumption is more likely to be 'ever not quite' in terms of an end goal of unification. Incompatibilities, differences of opinion, and a plurality of approaches which sometimes contradict and undermine each other are unproblematic from the perspective of accepting and tolerating dissensus (e.g. Rescher, 1993). (Issues around integration, common factors, and the concepts of weak and strong pluralism will be explored further in the next chapter, 'Common Factors'.)

In my view, much of the polarised discourses in the therapy field – around postmodernism/modernism, art/science, experience/evidence, as well as the pluralistic/monistic dimensions explored in this book – reflect a continuing reaction to the over-idealisation of the Enlightenment values of 'reason' and 'progress'. From William Blake onwards, the reductionist dangers of perceiving the world only through a scientific lens have been passionately challenged by various artists, philosophers, and theorists, up to the postmodernists and beyond. In that sense, it is nothing new, only now a scientistic culture is far more embedded and entrenched than it ever was in the 17th and 18th centuries. Those who do not necessarily want to privilege the art and craft of therapy over its scientific and evidence-based potentials but want them to be *included* still have many battles to fight. For instance, the famous Blake quote: 'I will not Reason & Compare: my business is to Create' (Blake, 1957/1804–1820, p. 629) is antithetical to how therapy situates itself and is situated in contemporary Western cultures.

The backlash against postmodernism is also propelled by a certain amount of misunderstanding and straw man arguments. For instance, Ellingham (2023) criticises Cooper and McLeod for being 'seduced by the half-truths of a philosophical movement termed "postmodernism": half-truths that have left them on a par with the person who says he both believes in God and is an atheist' (p. 4). This metaphor does not make sense, as postmodernists are more likely to say they cannot fully believe in either position without further unassailable evidence. In other words, a postmodernist position would most likely be one of agnosticism. Moreover, a postmodernist would not deny that both the theist and the atheist hold strong 'grand narratives' which hold greater or lesser degrees of influence, depending on historical and social contexts. Ellingham's critique of postmodernism is simultaneously influenced and contextualised by the contemporary and voguish trend to caricature postmodernism as a 'disaster' because of its scepticism towards and about 'liberal democracy' and 'Western civilization' (e.g. Pinker, 2019). In 2025, with wars raging as I write, these sacred cows seem less and less convincing. Perhaps a healthier, more pluralistic position is to move towards what some are calling metamodernism (e.g. Storm, 2021), in which the valid critiques of modernism by postmodernist theorists are not discarded but neither are worthwhile values contained in modernism and its antecedents in the Enlightenment. Storm also claims that this dialectical synthesis between modernism and postmodernism will evolve new ways of theorising and practising in various disciplines.

Concluding Thoughts

Both therapists and clients can have difficulties in understanding therapy as primarily about different approaches/techniques. The jury still appears to be out on whether transparency about different techniques/approaches is that helpful for clients, or even that relevant to practitioners. In a different vein, some practitioners and researchers call for an understanding of therapy that does not seek to understand what differentiates therapists and therapies from each other but, instead, what *common factors* lead to different therapists and therapies being effective. This view of therapy suggests that an ideal therapeutic world might be one in which therapy evolves to become one practice informed by the effective common factors of all therapies. This might be imagined as a potential diplomatic resolution to the debates about pluralism and therapy or, perhaps, an unnecessary homogenisation of creative differences. The next chapter focuses on the integrative drive for a unifying, if not quite unified, 'common factors' future for therapy and how the common factors agenda aligns, or does not align, with pluralism and pluralistic agendas for therapy.

Chapter 11

Common Factors and the Integrative Movement

Saul Rosenzweig

The idea that there are common factors in all therapies goes back to 1936 with the publication of Saul Rosenzweig's paper 'Some implicit common factors in diverse methods of psychotherapy: At last the Dodo said, "Everybody has won and all must have prizes"'(Rosenzweig, 1936). Research evidence which suggests that it is, indeed, the case that it is common factors which predict the efficaciousness of psychotherapy has come to be known as the 'Dodo effect' (e.g. Wampold & Imel, 2015). Rosenzweig argued that beneficial therapeutic factors might not be those which any given therapeutic theory postulates but less obvious common factors, such as the 'therapist's personality' (1936, p. 413), which might apply across a range of theories. To illustrate how far away the beneficial factors might be from those purposefully employed by the therapist, he suggested that a successful course of therapy with a psychoanalyst could be explained by Pavlovian behavioural changes rather than Freudian theory. While acknowledging that some approaches might be more effective with particular problems, Rosenzweig's view, on the whole, is that 'it is of comparatively little consequence what particular method [the] therapist uses' (p. 415). From a pluralistic perspective, it is also interesting to note that Rosenzweig suggested that the 'therapist should have a repertoire of methods to be drawn upon as needed for the individual case' (p. 415).

Jerome Frank

Frank's *Persuasion and Healing* (1961) suggested that common factors should not just be recognised in the relatively recent Western practice of therapy but for many healing practices across different cultures. Frank effectively created a common factors model, which Wampold and Imel (2015) acknowledge as the basis for their later Contextual Model. Frank argued that 'people seek psychotherapy for the demoralization that results from their symptoms rather than for symptom relief' (1961, p. 48). In other words, it is by engaging with the demoralisation rather than the 'depression', for instance, that makes therapy effective: a subtle but profound

DOI: 10.4324/9781003468332-11

differentiation to symptom-based models of research and practice. The main common factors that Frank and Frank (1991) identified are:

> [1] an *emotionally charged, confiding relationship with a helping person* ... [2] the context of the relationship is a *healing setting* ... [3] there exists a *rationale, conceptual scheme, or myth* that provides a plausible explanation for the patient's symptoms ... [and] [4] a *ritual or procedure* ... consistent with the rationale that was previously accepted by the client.
>
> (Wampold & Imel, 2015, p. 48, italics in original)

Bruce Wampold

The aforementioned Contextual Model, which Wampold developed with his student Zac Imel and others, holds that there are three pathways which 'contribute to the effects of psychotherapy' (Wampold, 2022). These are: 1) 'the caring, attentive, real and empathic relationship' 2) 'confidence in the treatment leads to expectations of change', and 3) 'the specific ingredients of the treatment'. These common factors can be looked at from four different 'levels of abstraction': 1) 'therapeutic techniques' (e.g. interpretations, chairwork), 2) 'therapeutic strategies' (e.g. collaboration, psychoeducation), 3) 'theoretical approaches' (e.g. person-centred, CBT), and 4) 'meta-theoretical models' (e.g. medical, contextual) (Wampold & Imel, 2015, p. 42).

Referring to the 'real relationship', Wampold suggests that '[t]he Contextual Model posits that the real relationship will be therapeutic in and of itself' (2015, p. 56). Regarding expectations, Wampold unapologetically connects this factor in successful therapy to the placebo effect and asserts that this is also true of 'many medical procedures' (2015, p. 57). In other words, if a placebo effect is operating in therapy, then that is as worthy of investigation and exploration as placebo factors in medicine and as valid, in terms of outcome. Wampold also suggests that the expectations which lead to placebo effects in therapy do not just occur randomly but are created in 'the interaction between the therapist and the client' (2015, p. 203). Finally, Wampold acknowledges the validity of specific ingredients, which, of course, might belong to specific, rather than all, approaches. However, in contrast to the medical model, Wampold suggests that his Contextual Model is concerned with specific ingredients, not to demonstrate the potency of a specific ingredient to ameliorate a specific 'deficit' but to demonstrate that whatever the specific ingredients they have the same effect of motivating the client 'to do something that is salubrious' (2015, p. 60).

Common factors are seen to be the cause of 'general effects'. The 'working alliance' is one aspect of the real relationship that is seen as vital to beneficial therapeutic outcomes (see also Clarkson, 2003/1995). Wampold (Wamplod & Imel, 2015) refers to Ed Bordin as defining the 'alliance between therapist and client' as a 'pan-theoretical construct consisting of three components: a) agreement about the goals of therapy; b) agreement about the tasks of therapy, and c) the bond between the therapist and client' (2015, p. 179). The terminology of goals and tasks aligns with Cooper's pluralistic therapy framework, as does the language of Hatcher and Barends (2006), who define the alliance as 'the degree to which the therapy dyad is engaged in collaborative, purposive work (p. 293)' (cited in Wampold & Imel, 2015, p. 179).

Wampold's Contextual Model has been subject to some critiques, noticeably by Lars-Gunnar Lundh (2014). He names the common factors models of both Frank and Wampold as Relational-Procedural Persuasion (RPP) models and, in contrast to these models, proposes a Methodological Principles and Skills (MPS) model. He differentiates the MPS model from the RPP model because it is only the former model, he claims, which assumes that 'effective psychotherapy relies on common methodological principles' and that 'method matters' (p. 131). Lundh also claims that 'it is possible to improve existing methods' (p. 131). Lundh proposed his model in the *Psychology and Behavioral Sciences* journal, so, unsurprisingly, he assumes that therapy is, and should be, perceived as a behavioural science. He recognises that Frank and Frank do not. This is illustrative of the art/science debate referred to throughout this book, with implications about modern and postmodern sensibilities referred to in the previous chapter. He also recognises that Wampold's Contextual Model is an explicit challenge to the medical model, similarly illustrating the medical/non-medical conceptualisations of therapy.

Lundh suggests that as well as common relational factors there are also '*methodological commonalities*' (2014, p. 132), such as corrective experiences, therapist feedback, exposure, and emotional processing. He discerns methodological principles in Frank and Frank's model – such as emotional arousal – and states that their model can therefore be seen as a mixture of RPP and MPS models in contrast to Wampold's Contextual Model, which is a 'pure' RPP model (because it only acknowledges the effects of particular methods as due to their nature as rituals, adhering to previously accepted myths and rationales rather than being due to the methods themselves).

In general terms, Lundh associates his conception of an MPS model with integrative theorists such as Goldfried. The latter conceptualises therapy as operating on 'three levels of abstraction: (1) theoretical models, (2) methodological principles, and (3) specific techniques' (2014, p. 136). Goldfried suggests that common factors are mostly found at the second level as principles 'like the provision of a new view of self, the establishment of a working alliance, and the facilitation of corrective experiences' (p. 136).

There is a certain amount of fear in Lundh's paper that without the integration of his MPS model with the RRP model psychotherapy might not be recognised as having any real effect. In other words, since the common factors can apply to other healing relationships, there is nothing unique or special about psychotherapy. From a pluralistic perspective, this is unthreatening. The possibility that therapy might be one healing process in a family of healing processes does not lessen the value of therapy as a modern healing practice. It offers myths, rationales, and procedures that resonate more with contemporary people than, say, shamanism. There are those, even within our own conventional cultures, who might prefer to see a shaman rather than a therapist, and if that works for them, from a pluralistic perspective, that is wholly unproblematic. However, Lundh questions that if psychotherapy really is akin to other healing practices then the costly trainings associated with it might not be justified. This, to me, is a separate issue. Training costs are associated with the time and energy put into learning, which might be even greater in, say, shamanism. Yet Lundh insists that it is imperative that there are psychotherapy-specific, method-based factors with a scientific basis to justify psychotherapy in the 'Western' world (again, illustrating a science/art division). How much time and energy needs to be spent in attaining some kind of level sanctioned by others is a debate which I have explored in previous chapters and will explore further in the next chapter in relation to issues around professionalisation and regulation.

Common Factors and the Integrative Movement

There is a kind of split within both the profession and researchers, between those who advocate that there are better and worse approaches (in themselves and excluding *other factors*) and those who are more sympathetic to the idea that perhaps it is not the approach that matters so much as those *other factors*. In research based on the medical model, it is, in fact, imperative to identify specific factors rather than non-specific common factors (e.g. Butler & Strupp, 1986), which from a scientific perspective are merely 'placebo', as discussed previously.

The idea of common factors aligns with emphasising the importance of process as much as outcome, and so researchers interested in trying to determine the generic ingredients of successful practice emphasise process factors, and research suggests that some generic process factors such as 'hope, expectation, relationship with the therapist, belief, and corrective experience' (Wampold & Imel, 2015, p. 33) are associated with positive outcomes but not aligned to any particular approach.

A pluralistic approach, in my view, does not need to have quite the same agenda as those pushing for integrative/common factors approaches to research and practice, but it does share the same goal of trying to encourage different ways of practising, supported by research (e.g. Cooper & McLeod, 2011; Norcross & Goldfried, 2005).

The integrative movement as a whole was based on 'dissatisfaction with individual theoretical approaches' (Wampold & Imel, 2015, p. 45). Within the integrative movement, Arkowitz (1992) identified three distinct pathways towards integration: 1) theoretical integration, 2) technical eclecticism, and 3) common factors. Theoretical integration 'is the fusion of two or more theories into a single conceptualization' (Wampold & Imel, 2015, p. 46); technical eclecticism attempts to tailor therapeutic approaches and techniques by considering the specifics of clients, therapists, and problems; and the common factors approach 'attempts to identify and codify the aspects of therapy common to all psychotherapies' (Wampold & Imel, 2015, p. 47). A fourth pathway, 'assimilative integration', is another pathway towards therapy integration 'in which therapists gradually introduce new techniques and ideas into their pre-existing approach' (Cooper & McLeod, 2011, p. 5). Since 2019, the *Journal of Psychotherapy Integration* (*JPI*), a publication for the Society for the Exploration of Psychotherapy Integration (SEPI), has identified a fifth pathway of integration – unification – described as 'meta-theoretical approaches which place theories, techniques, and principles into holistic frameworks' (see the *JPI* website and Marquis, 2024).

From a pluralistic standpoint, theoretical integration ultimately just creates another singular model that can be used by therapists and clients (or not), depending on preference. So, it fits into a pluralistic view as just one more approach. Technical eclecticism is not the same as, but is very similar to, pluralistic therapy: some argue pluralistic therapy is just technical eclecticism under a different banner (e.g. Ellingham, 2023). This can be refuted by emphasising that central features of pluralistic therapy are collaboration (e.g. McLeod, 2018) and a deep valuing of the other (e.g. Cooper, 2024b), which are not necessary preconditions for practising from a technical eclectic position. However, despite those differences, it is still too close to a pluralistic perspective on therapy to be seen as significantly different. Similarly, assimilative integration holds a liberal view regarding the practitioner adapting an approach but does not depart significantly from it and so, arguably, remains singular. In some ways, the concept of unification as an integrative pathway describes pluralistic therapy when it emphasises its utility as a framework. However, this is somewhat muddled by the latter's claim to also being a coherent and singular approach, particularly in its ambitions to be codified enough for trainings and research. This holding on to being both a framework and a codified practice is at least theoretically problematic, as pointed out throughout this book.

The common factors and unification integrative pathways, arguably, contrast most markedly with pluralism. A common factors view of therapy is less about adhering to an approach and more about trying to identify and create generic qualities of practice which might apply to any approach. Norcross and Saltzman (1990) recognise '*common-factor approaches*' as one of few attempts contributing towards 'the contemporary movement to integrate the psychotherapies' (p. 3, italics in original). Most therapists would agree that therapies have at least some common factors, even if they want to claim that their particular approach also contains factors which make theirs better or different. With regards to unification, some pluralist theorists conceptualise a pluralism which envisages Many within a One ('e pluribus unum'), but even therapy integrationists admit that a unified therapy field is a somewhat distant dream. Furthermore, it is debatable whether unification is actually an ideal worth progressing towards. Many therapy integrationists assume that gaining thus far unattained scientific credibility for the therapy field is of the utmost importance, when, arguably, they are committing an egregious category error in insisting on therapy as needing to fit into an overarching scientific paradigm.

The common factors and unification approaches figure most prominently as a counterpoint to a pluralistically informed perspective. This will be explored in more detail in a subsequent section after a brief exploration of different therapeutic approaches as different languages.

Therapeutic Approaches as Languages

The integrative movement has provided strong arguments that align with some pluralistic attitudes and insights. Importantly, it was early to critique the therapeutic field by suggesting that many therapies have different names for the same thing. Miller, Duncan and Hubble's *Escape from Babel* (1997), which sought to create a 'unifying language for psychotherapy practice', illustrated how therapeutic orientations sometimes struggle to distinguish themselves from each other yet still insist on doing so for political and economic reasons. In contrast, the authors claim that 'words are practically all that separates the models from each other' (p. 11).

Goodman (2016) also suggests that different therapeutic orientations are 'actually different languages that human beings have for understanding their suffering, meaning, identity, and healing' (p. 80). He warns that the limited availability of different types of therapy, particularly for those on lower incomes, could lead to '"therapy deserts" comparable to "food deserts"'(p. 86), in which individuals can only access '*processed psychotherapies*' (italics in original) which only have '[miniscule] language variations' (p. 86). He suggests that this has arisen because of the 'McDonaldization of Society' (e.g. Ritzer, 2015), in which the values of '*predictability, control, calculability,* and *efficiency*' (Goodman, 2016, p. 89; italics in original) uncritically dominate decision-making.

So, if different therapeutic perspectives are like different languages: psychodynamic language, CBT language, person-centred language, TA language, and so forth, then, in this conception, as long as both client and therapist are happy to be talking in that language, a therapeutic relationship can evolve, especially if the dialogical aspect of using the language is understood as including all aspects of communications and not just what might be textually transcribed. If the client and therapist are not 'talking the same language' or do not want to, then a referral onwards would be advised. The issue is not so much about the client or the therapist but about the language they use to symbolise their perspectives on reality in their interaction (in their *symbolic interaction* – see, e.g., Scott, 2015).

These different therapy languages can be pragmatically *used*, much like a human being can speak a language while not necessarily having any deep connection to the culture that produced it. This conceptualisation can lead in either pluralistic or integrative directions – on that level, pluralism and integration might be seen as sharing common ground.

If different therapies are more like different languages, rather than truly inhabiting any significantly different processual realities, then it follows that what some defend as being different phenomena are actually only different word/name symbolisations for the same phenomena, and this acts as a basis and argument for an integrative and common factors approach.

Similarities between apparently different approaches and theories in therapy include TA's concept of the 'script' and narrative therapy (e.g. Gilbert & Orlans, 2011). Additionally, Eric Berne conceptualised the idea of the Child ego state in the early 1960s, which is much the same idea as the 'inner child' popularised by

many others from the 1970s onwards (e.g. Bradshaw, 2024/1990) and also elaborated further in the currently fashionable Internal Family Systems approach (e.g.
Schwarz, 1995).

In a similar vein, it might be argued that Cooper and McLeod's version of pluralistic therapy is an attempt to build a vocabulary more than an approach to enable
the concepts embedded in the vocabulary to be valid enough to undergo 'scientific'
testing.

Pluralism and Integrationism: The Same or Different?

Whether pluralistic therapy – or pluralism held as a philosophical basis for practice
– aligns with integration is a point of contention and confusion amongst theorists.
For instance, in much of the literature, the terms 'integrative' and 'pluralistic' are
often confounded so readers might assume they are one and the same. Some pluralistic theorists (e.g. McLeod, 2018) put pluralistic therapy under the integrative umbrella. This suggests that the Many can be included in an idealised One. Following
James, the prospect of attaining a 'One' for therapy, or indeed other phenomena,
is 'ever not quite' (Araujo & Osbeck, 2023). From this angle, what can distinguish
pluralistic therapy more philosophically and politically is to conceptualise pluralistic therapy as uncommitted to integrative ambitions or ideals – the purpose of a
pluralistically-informed therapy being that differences, boundaries, and multiplicity are perceived as fundamentally unproblematic, or if not unproblematic, at least
a reality that needs to be accepted.

In contrast, some integrationists and common factors theorists are quite open
that their ambition is to ultimately create a unified field for therapy (e.g. Marquis,
2024; Kramer, 2024). The common factors movement might, in future, form the
basis of a research-based and/or evidence-based generic therapy in which distinct
models lose their importance. On that level, although the ideal of unification is not
any immediate threat, there are some potential dangers in the over-idealisation of
integration and the search for common factors.

Marquis (2024) describes the 'framing' of common factors 'within a unified
metatheory', suggesting that

> unifying frameworks [it is worth noting that the emphasis is on frameworks
> rather than approaches] allow us to coherently order and conceptualize the
> abundance of phenomena relevant to psychotherapy, the methods with which
> we study those phenomena, and how we apply such knowledge to the practice
> and training of psychotherapy.
>
> (p. 213)

He suggests that although unification may be some way off, it is the only way
for the therapy field to evolve even if the ideal of unification is more of a process
than an endpoint (similar to how McLennan views pluralism as 'a way of seeing,

rather than a substantive "end-point" doctrine to believe in' (1995, p. ix)). This conclusion is reached via the assumption that not attempting processes of unification will hinder progress in the field. This underlying spirit of the unification agenda goes against, for instance, William Blake's assertion that 'Without Contraries is no progression' (Blake, 1957/1790–1793, p. 149). It is also assumed that consensus is crucial, as opposed to pluralistic thinking, which eschews the demand for consensus (e.g. Rescher, 1993). However, Marquis insists that the unification agenda 'is not incompatible with theoretical and methodological diversity and pluralism' (Marquis, 2024, p. 214) and is not against pluralism.

Marquis sees the contemporary therapy field as 'in a state of fragmented pluralism' (2024, p. 215). Despite his assurances that unification is not against pluralism, the easy association of fragmentation (used pejoratively) with pluralism demonstrates some ambivalence and, perhaps, some further association of pluralism with postmodern sensibilities (as discussed in the previous chapter), which might not have the same faith in science as a potential saviour for the credibility and success of therapy.

Ultimately, like Ellingham (2023), the basic complaint is that the therapy field is 'preparadigmatic' and is, therefore, not a 'mature discipline' (Marquis, 2024, p. 215). According to Marquis, it is only on the basis of unified assumptions and 'sound scientific evidence' that the therapy field can gain the ideal status of a mature discipline, notwithstanding that what therapy might need more than maturation is a major paradigm shift. Those who embrace unification tend to speak medical model language and uncritically use terms like 'assessment', 'case conceptualization', 'treatment plan', and 'evidence-based practice' (p. 215). The assumption that therapy needs to be a science alongside implicit bias against an art/praxis view of therapy sets up the possibility for a unifying therapy but one with a scientistic bent, which paradoxically cannot include all practitioners.

In similar ways to unification as an integrative pathway, Cooper and McLeod's agenda for their version of pluralistic therapy to be researched with a distinct emphasis on outcomes also blurs the philosophical bases of pluralism. The conceptualisation of helpful factors and processes (e.g. Antoniou et al., 2017) and the focus on identifying these helpful factors and processes for particular client groups or identifying methods that might be of use to the pluralistic therapist come close to being indistinguishable from the more established common factors theoretical and practice-based research (e.g. Hubble et al., 1999). It is not clear whether Cooper and McLeod envision, in the end, a more generic, integrated future for therapy with a base of 'evidence' for particular interventions or a pluralistic future for therapies. They might see this view as falling into the trap of either/or thinking, but the difference between a unified, integrated, generic 'therapy' and a plurality of 'therapies' could be said to represent opposite ends of a continuum of how therapy is theorised and practised, and might be theorised and practised. The research they have produced or encouraged – and the flexibility of their definitions of a 'pluralistic' approach – supports the view of some critics that their approach lacks philosophical coherence and integrity. Some research on the pluralistic framework seems to have just one pragmatic aim: proving itself to potential providers.

McLeod (2018) argues that the purist/integrative binary is unhelpful and erroneous. So-called 'pure' models, for example, are themselves usually integrations of various 'ideas and methods that were in circulation at the time they were founded' (p. 21). He also points out the commercial implications of tangible models versus practitioners just practising, who are not motivated to take their ideas 'to market'. The idea that 'all therapy is one thing' (p. 22) is also referred to, which, if true, has implications for therapy being pluralistic and points to accepting a more common factors view. Likewise, Cooper and McLeod (e.g. 2011) have also attempted to differentiate their pluralistic therapy by referring to it as a 'meta-model of therapy integration' (McLeod & Sundet, 2016, p. 160). This fudges the distinction between pluralism and integration, avoiding profound philosophical and political differences.

McLennan (1995) suggested that the boundary of pluralism might be considered to be integration: pluralism celebrates difference and wants to retain diversity, whereas integration wishes to homogenise multiplicity into unity. It could be argued that the implicit ideal of the integrationists, particularly the common factors integrationists, is to create a therapy that is called one thing, whether that be 'counselling', 'therapy', 'psychotherapy', or 'psychological therapy', and within that one thing practitioners would use the common factors of many therapies that are all, in some way, rooted in 'evidence'. A pluralistic attitude would defend the separate identities of different therapies as holistic, irreducible processes in which the need to identify and 'prove' the efficiency of sub-processual elements is possible but unnecessary.

Ultimately, it seems as if Cooper and McLeod support a more integrationist perspective, albeit wanting the integrative movement to take on a more pluralistic perspective (e.g. Cooper, 2019a). If this is the case, then the pluralistic philosophical basis of their pragmatic pluralistic project fades, and it becomes more challenging to see substantial philosophical and political differences between their aims and those of integrationists. This is not to criticise the common factors and integrative movements in themselves. From a pluralistic perspective, the theories and practices found within both common factors and integrative approaches have much to offer a pluralistic view of therapy. Rather, it is to criticise the notion that the pluralistic nature of the psychotherapeutic field (in terms of a multiplicity of sometimes irreconcilable theories and practices) is problematic and that similarities must be privileged over differences to facilitate a unified field. From a pluralistic perspective, diversification and difference are to be celebrated despite potential difficulties or problems.

Blunden (2024) conceptualises a 'pluralistic integration' (p. 214) process in elucidating what she means by pluralistic person-centred therapy. She makes an important distinction by describing pluralistic integration as 'a dialogical response to the unique needs and wishes of the client' versus a 'pre-existing framework' (p. 214).

This conception of an integrative therapy (which is always in a process of 'becoming' rather than 'fixed') being created in dialogue *with* rather than theorising *over* is a way of conceptualising integration that reflects a pluralistic philosophy and practice. Blunden differentiates this kind of pluralistic integration from integrative approaches, which are 'synthesising' (see theoretical integration), and the 'eclectic form' (e.g. technical eclecticism) thus:

> Both the synthesising and eclectic forms of integration effectively place the design of the therapeutic approach into the hands of the therapist ... Pluralistic integration, by contrast, places responsibility for the integrative design of the therapy on the co-productive therapeutic relationship ... the structure of therapy is mutually discovered by the therapist and client in real time ... carefully and systematically sharing the integrative design process with clients, according to their needs and inclinations ...
>
> (p. 215)

Brown and Smith (2023) similarly claim this pluralistic integration process as a basis for pluralistic practice more broadly and state that it is an 'integrative approach ... unique in the way integration happens' (p. 15).

Concluding Thoughts

Overall, the common factors perspective offers hopeful ground on which pluralistic attitudes to therapy might flourish. Research evidence supports the notion that what makes therapy effective is not particular approaches but common factors (e.g. Wampold & Imel, 2015). A practice based on applying and acknowledging common factors offers a 'non-denominational' route for those who do not want to identify with particular approaches but, instead, want to engage with effective therapeutic practices from different approaches.

If common factors research were to be more fully acknowledged and respected, the rationale for comparing the effectiveness of approaches against each other would soon collapse (2015). Research should focus on more relevant factors of therapeutic effectiveness, such as the processual elements of clients, therapists, and their relationships.

Pluralistic therapists need to assume the importance of common factors. However, this does not mean that recognising common factors needs to lead to generic forms of therapy subservient to 'evidence-based' approaches or even evidence-based micro-processual 'interventions'. The recognition of common factors which simultaneously allows for a multiplicity of approaches to flourish more accurately reflects a pluralistic position.

Recognising that different therapeutic approaches might be effective *because of* common factors could mitigate the threat of future practitioners who choose not to use empirically validated treatments being further marginalised or, worse, perceived as practising unethically (e.g. Bryceland & Stam, 2018; Goodman, 2016).

Contemporary and historical understandings of therapy as more rooted in similarities than differences need to be protected and promoted.

Some theorists also suggest that 'efforts to unify ... under a single conceptual scheme' (Araujo & Osbeck, 2023, p. 27) and the dangers of 'homogenization' (p. 27) thereof might be solved by a dialectical pluralism (Goertzen, 2010) 'consisting of a back and forth, dialogical relationship between different phases of pluralism: convergent pluralism, in which the emphasis is on integration ... and divergent pluralism, wherein the limits of integration are explored' (Araujo & Osbeck, 2023, p. 27). This would allow for the possibilities of integration and aiming for the One while holding that there is also value in accepting plurality, difference, and the Many. Not only the Many (therapies) which have already been established but the Many (therapies) constantly being created and innovated, such as Blunden's tailored integrations in each and every therapeutic relationship.

Chapter 12

Pluralism and the Future of Therapy

Professionalisation and Regulation

In the gradual professionalisation of therapy, there has been a steadily increasing demand for different types of regulation, with some demanding that there needs to be statutory regulation (SR) sooner rather than later. One of the main rationales behind the demand for SR is that it will protect the public from dangerous therapists (e.g. Hall, 2024a; 2024b). We explored the history of the moves towards regulation in Chapter 2, and the pressure for SR continues, most recently since the election of a Labour government in the UK in 2024.

Often, critics of the regulatory systems which are already in place suggest that the therapy professions are not regulated at all. However, this is a false allegation as they are regulated, just not by the State – through ethics and standards to which they are expected to conform by their professional bodies under the umbrella of the Professional Standards Authority for Health and Social Care (PSA). The hope of those pushing for SR is that the protection of titles such as 'counsellor' and 'psychotherapist' will mean that less harm is likely to occur since this protection will allow practitioners to be struck off regulated registers. They can already be, and often are, struck off regulated registers. The apparently important difference with SR is that continuing to practise with a title after being struck off becomes a criminal offence, which it is not currently. However, the sticky problem of bad actors – practising either without the necessary qualifications in the first place or having been struck off with them – simply taking on different unregulated titles such as 'anxiety coach' or 'trauma expert', or a multitude of other easily-invented titles, is never answered. Nor is the problem of established mental health providers such as the NHS inventing a plethora of new titles such as 'psychological wellbeing practitioner', to enable staff to practise with less formal training (and associated lower salaries).

The central assumption which comes into play when making demands for therapy to be statutorily regulated is that therapy is a healthcare profession (e.g. Hall, 2024b). This assumption has been challenged throughout this book, and there are dangers in any regulations that assume therapy is a medical activity rather than a relational one. One danger is that statutory regulators are responsible for,

DOI: 10.4324/9781003468332-12

amongst other responsibilities, the educational and training requirements for entry to a profession. This is likely to increase costs for practitioners, create barriers to entry in a profession already heavily critiqued for its financial and class elitism, and, just as importantly, standardise and homogenise the pluralistic possibilities of therapy which otherwise might be more innovative, more creative, and able to offer a multitude of therapies for a multitude of different types of people with different needs and wants. Moreover, unfortunately, the NHS and NICE's history in shaping how therapy is provided does not suggest that state regulators will have a sympathetic and understanding grasp of therapy's potential to help those in distress.

The strongest objections to SR come from the Alliance for Counselling and Psychotherapy (ACP). This organisation successfully contributed to stopping SR in the period leading up to the election of a Conservative government in 2010. And now the call for SR is resurfacing; with the election of a new government and media pressure concerning disturbing stories of therapist abuse, they are revitalising their campaign against it because of the same concerns they had from 2006 onwards. They argue that since egregious offences are committed by statutorily regulated professions, the common perception that SR will protect the public is not valid. Pro-SR practitioners also imagine SR will lead to more job opportunities and professional respect, especially within publicly-funded providers such as the NHS. The ACP refutes this and thinks that energy might be more usefully directed at more successfully communicating to the public and providers about the benefits of therapy and how it might be even more beneficial if there was meaningful choice for clients/patients. They acknowledge that the system in place might be improved but do not see SR as the 'way forward' and, instead, suggest that there be a national conference for all interested parties to have an open and, hopefully, fruitful dialogue (ACP, 2024).

Currently, in the UK, therapy is regulated by the PSA. The present UK government suggests that this system is a 'proportionate means of assurance for unregulated professions, that sits between employer controls and statutory regulation by setting standards for organisations holding voluntary registers' (Department of Health and Social Care, 2024). Although this system is not perfect, the ACP suggests it is 'the "least worst" system' (ACP, 2024).

So, for now, the impact of professionalisation and regulation on the therapy professions is in a kind of holding pattern, but that could change, and those interested in a pluralistic attitude towards therapy provision need to be aware of how different moves towards SR may or may not impact the profession. The most significant change in the UK has been the evolution of the Scope of Practice and Education framework (SCoPEd) from a 'mapping exercise' to something which is being implemented by most major counselling and psychotherapy organisations (accredited by the PSA). Although SCoPEd has not been explicitly connected to the SR agenda, it is implicitly suggested, as it could quell debates about definitions of therapy, which is a prerequisite for statutory regulation. This will be further explored in the next section.

The Scope of Practice and Education Framework (SCoPEd)

The main attempt to further professionalise and regulate the therapeutic professions within the UK has been via the controversial SCoPEd project. Rather than working towards a common entry point for both counsellors and psychotherapists or a system in which a variety of qualifications and specialisms are recognised, the SCoPEd project instead emphasises initial trainings in what seems like an attempt to institutionalise an apparent superiority for 'psychotherapists' (column C in the current version) over and above column B and column A 'counsellors'. The system is unapologetically hierarchical.

The main impact of this seems to be on courses and trainings, which are adapting their syllabuses and delivery models to ensure as much as possible that their training programmes are further up the hierarchy, then promising in advertising and so forth what column their graduates will be able to claim post-qualification. Additionally, for already qualified therapists who have been blindsided by SCoPEd (despite warnings from some in the profession), new add-on trainings are being marketed to enable them to gain as high a place as possible in the new hierarchy. BACP practitioners in column A (some with decades of experience and multiple trainings) need to spend time and money on the BACP accreditation scheme (formerly a voluntary 'badge' that many practitioners neither wanted nor needed) to gain column B or column C status. Furthermore, thus far, there are no 'grandparenting' schemes for those who have already attained 'senior accredited' status within the BACP to be approved for column C more easily. Similar issues exist for other membership bodies accredited by the PSA (such as the Association of Christian Counsellors, the Human Givens Institute, and the NCPS). The only therapists in the major counselling and psychotherapy membership bodies who remain detrimentally unaffected by the new categorisations are 'psychotherapists' recognised as such by the BPC and the UKCP. Significantly, some PSA-accredited registers, such as the CBT Register and COSCA (Counselling and Psychotherapy in Scotland), are not aligning their qualifications with the SCoPEd framework.

A major criticism of SCoPEd is that it seems to unquestioningly favour practitioners who work from a medical model perspective, even though many therapists purposefully and ethically want to work with whole persons rather than part symptoms. From a pluralistic perspective, this diminishment of relational therapy over instrumental, diagnostically-based models endangers therapies which do not conform to the hegemonic worldviews being privileged within medicalised systems. Other issues in relation to the medical model's continuing influence in the therapy field are explored in the next section.

Many practitioners have flagged up various controversial issues around SCoPEd from its conception. The membership bodies only superficially dealt with innovative and creative ideas about how it might be adapted or changed to avoid such issues. It was a project led mainly from the top without much input from those working on the front lines in everyday practices or the training and education of therapists. In addition, it was initially sold as a 'mapping exercise' and, perhaps predictably, soon became an action plan that therapists, trainers, and educators now must engage with to align with the membership bodies' new vision for therapy. What was an idea is now becoming a new reality with implications for the pluralistic future of therapy, for similar reasons to the issues around professionalisation and regulation more generally.

All these issues relate to the troubled relationship of therapy with the medical model explored throughout this book and briefly recapped in the next section.

The Medical Model

Issues around therapy being or not being aligned with the medical model are closely related to the professionalisation and regulation of therapy. Therapy, rightly or wrongly, is often associated with the medical model, and medicalising distress is often, if not always, problematic and potentially harmful (e.g. Linder, 2024). Therapists in the USA are, arguably, even more aligned to the medical model than their colleagues in the UK because of the emphasis on the medical model in trainings and, specifically, because so many people access therapists via medical insurance schemes. The parallel to this in the UK is the NHS, and there are inevitable differences in interests and practices between private, independent practitioners and those working for the NHS. So much so that those who align with the medical model, either personally or via training or approach, are privileged within that system. Indeed, the NHS continues to create its own therapy trainings to fit into its system rather than include therapists and attempt to understand how and why they train and qualify in ways developed over more than a century and how and why they continue to remain in demand outside the NHS if not within it.

The medical paradigm for mental health has been subject to critique over many years, and the call for a more person-centred (in the broad meaning of the term) approach to mental health care across the world continues. This call, far from being a fringe view, as it might have been when Szasz published his seminal *The Myth of Mental Illness* (1961), is becoming increasingly mainstream and supported by many mental health professionals (e.g. Poole, 2024). A non-medicalised approach would also benefit a plurality of therapies and a plurality of different types of people with problems in living.

Pluralism(s): Philosophy, Politics, Practice

Following Araujo and Osbeck (2023), the starting point for understanding the implications of pluralism for therapy is the recognition that there is a plurality of types of pluralism and the multitude of different meanings it has depending on context and intentions. Cooper's pluralism is increasingly informed by the relational ethics of Levinas, in which ontologies, epistemologies, and methodologies are not seen as important as ethics and, in particular, the fundamental ethic of caring (e.g. Cooper, 2024b). This is in contrast to a Jamesian pluralism, which is more comprehensive and attempts to understand the implications of pluralism applied to those areas which Levinasian pluralism demotes. Cooper also favours a pluralism in which a multitude of positions can be grounded in a 'singular set of values' (Cooper, 2019b). This grasping for a One in which to contain the Many is certainly a type of pluralism which some call moderate, weak, or reasonable pluralism. Assuming a moderate pluralistic position avoids the accusation of understanding pluralism as meaning 'anything goes', to which stronger takes on pluralism are more vulnerable. However, at the same time, it, more problematically, also avoids the realities of irreconcilable differences and what some call the 'problem of pluralism' (e.g. Lassman, 2011). The fact of pluralism (Lassman, 2011) and associated problems of fundamental but reasonable disagreements means that various areas of human activities, usually identified as political but easily applied to therapy, need to admit that agreements cannot always be found. The acceptance of this problem is, in fact, paradoxically, the first step towards ameliorating it. It is a democratic principle that because unification is, in effect, an ideal rather than any imminent reality, we need to learn to live with disagreements rather than wishing them away. With this view in mind and applied to the field of therapy, it might be suggested that all the opposing positions (theoretical, practical, political) are not something to be appeased by an appeal to some mollifying unity but, rather, the dissensus is something to be accepted and worked with as a worthwhile struggle.

Pluralistic Therapy

In this sub-section, the future of Cooper and McLeod's pluralistic therapy, in particular, will be explored. A principal aim of this book has been to demonstrate that the philosophies and politics of pluralism(s) can be used as lenses with which to view therapy as a whole and specific domains within it, without any need to identify as a pluralistic practitioner. However, inarguably, many of the innovations in theorising how pluralism might relate to therapeutic practices have come from Cooper and McLeod and their associates. Their version of pluralistic therapy (and their ongoing articulations, conceptualisations, and networking initiatives around it) remains a vital resource for considering the relationship between pluralism and therapy. For some, the actual framework and approach (the protocolled practice versus a looser perspective) might be all that is needed and wanted in order to incorporate a pluralistic take on therapy. In that sense, it is central to the future of pluralistic ideas applied to therapy, and therefore the rest of this section will explore the future of their pluralistic therapy in and on its own terms.

One significant development in pluralistic therapy has been its increasingly political stances as connected to pluralistic implications for therapy. Cooper (2024c) has recently asserted that the 'pluralistic approach to therapy is grounded in principles of progressive social change' (p. 1). By progressive social change, Cooper means not just believing in the concept and importance of social justice but also believing that social justice can be realised in the future. Within the concept of progressive social change, there is also the wish to maximise as well as equalise human potential (Cooper, 2024c). Furthermore, in a post-humanistic spirit, in which humanism might be criticised for being too anthropocentric, progressive social change, of course, includes concerns for animals and the environment as well as human beings (2024c). Essentially, Cooper continues to develop his ideas around the synergy between progressive social change perspectives and therapy, first extensively explored and theorised in *Psychology at the Heart of Social Change* (Cooper, 2023).

The love of forms and feedback measures also continues within the pluralistic therapy approach. Cooper claims that 'pluralistic therapy ... encourages routine outcome monitoring ... as a means of accessing and amplifying the experience of the client' (Cooper, 2024c, p. 13). The critiques of such somewhat bureaucratic monitoring as reflecting a wider audit culture and scientism, as discussed previously, are acknowledged but ignored. Where this puts therapists who resonate with a more pluralistic attitude towards therapy but who are simultaneously uncomfortable with interrupting the flow of sessions with the use of forms is unclear.

In 2024, the central figures promoting pluralistic therapy launched an open-access journal called *Pluralistic Practice*. This journal extends the idea of pluralistic practice from therapy into other fields. It aims to:

> [support] the development of a global community of inquiry within which practitioners, communities, and citizens can share knowledge, experience, and evidence around the challenges and benefits of working pluralistically to facilitate individual and collective well-being, solidarity, and justice.
>
> (Blunden et al., 2024)

This call for an interdisciplinary approach to pluralism and the possibilities of pluralistic principles being applied to practice in various disciplines is a positive development, and it will be interesting to see how the journal fares over the coming years.

Pluralistic Therapy and the Person-Centred Approach (PCA)

Debates about whether pluralistic therapy has any right to claim any territory of person-centred theory and practice will inevitably continue. This is a relatively new development as, in the original iterations of pluralistic therapy (although roots in humanistic–existential ethics were acknowledged), Cooper, McLeod and others did not specify pluralistic therapy as a 'tribe' of person-centred therapy. This has irked some in the person-centred community, as it is not that they have anything against pluralistic therapy *per se* (mostly), but, as previously mentioned, they do object to what is perceived as an unnecessary encroachment of person-centred practice. They also suggest that pluralistic theorists distort the meanings of the PCA through misunderstandings of what it means to be person-centred. For many person-centred practitioners, the *sine qua non* of person-centred practice is a belief in the actualising tendency (e.g. Molyneux, 2024). Molyneux also asserts that the six conditions must also be believed to be a necessary foundation for any practice defining itself as person-centred.

Although how pluralistic therapy might be applied to different therapeutic approaches was articulated in *The Handbook of Pluralistic Counselling and Psychotherapy* (Cooper & Dryden, 2016), there was no attempt to merge it directly with any particular approaches. And, in any case, to want to do so seems to be going against a pluralistic spirit. Yet, there is a growing movement of therapists identifying as person-centred but with a pluralistic take on the approach – a Venn diagram intersection where pluralistic therapy and person-centred therapy meet.

To my mind, person-centred therapy, whether it is practised purely or not, is philosophically and practically pluralistic. By this, I mean that because it is ideally client-led, so that the therapist responds to the client, then it will, therefore, proceed in potentially infinite directions, unlike a manualised or protocolled therapy, which is necessarily constrained. This does not mean, however, that it *is* pluralistic therapy. It is its own thing, which from a pluralistic philosophical position needs to be accepted as a valid single approach whether one agrees or disagrees with its assumptions.

There is a useful distinction to be made between Rogerian and post-Rogerian person-centred theory as applied to therapeutic practice versus person-centred approaches as applied in healthcare and other sectors (e.g. Skills for Health, 2017). The latter emphasises person-centredness along similar lines to how pluralistic therapists and theorists define their conceptions of the core values of the PCA, especially the emphasis on collaboration. A way forward might be to redefine the pluralistic/person-centred interface as one allying itself with the broader meanings of person-centred rather than Rogerian and post-Rogerian person-centred practices more specifically.

Artificial Intelligence (AI)

Political and philosophical issues continue to cause divisions in the therapy field, and how they are or are not resolved will determine the future of therapy. Alongside these issues, which, though various and changing, have been constant since Freud, AI is the most recent external development that will impact the future of therapy for both the profession and the people it serves in this digital era. And, as with other areas of human life, the impact will inevitably have positive and negative consequences.

AI Therapy (AIT) and 'chatbot therapists' (e.g. Robb, 2024) are already here. There are 'around 10,000 apps or chatbots that can give you free, or extremely cheap, 24/7 mental health support' and the 'mental health app market is forecast to be worth £13.8 billion by 2030' (Ford, 2024). Therapy 'as an open, person-to-person, encounter is becoming the privilege of the few who can afford professional fees' (Atkinson, 2024, p. 1). Atkinson contrasts this kind of therapy with behavioural therapy, the usual NHS offer. He predicts that, for most people, behavioural therapy, not just in the UK but around the world, 'will be conducted by machine and algorithm' (p. 1). The NHS is, indeed, already integrating AIT via apps such as Wysa (p. 2). The ideal of AIT is to create sophisticated 'conversational agents' (CAs) which will, via the 'technology that integrates artificial intelligence, natural language processing (NLP), and machine learning (ML) ... make chatbots smarter and capable of having more human-like conversations' (p. 2). Much of the data for improving the interactions with clients comes from the NHS, from text exchanges between therapists and clients (Atkinson, 2024, p. 3) as well as session recordings.

Potential advantages of AIT include: 1) it can reach far more people than in-person therapy, 2) it is cheaper, 3) it can act as a first step towards in-person therapy, 4) it is available twenty-four hours a day, and 5) it is accessible via a smartphone (e.g. Michele, 2024). All these features mean that public sector health providers such as the NHS can offer more mental health support.

However, there are disadvantages. Most concerning is the fact that AI, in order to emulate the characteristics of therapy sessions, needs to utilise the data of actual sessions. This data is provided by recorded and/or transcribed sessions and/ or summaries of sessions. If held on servers, these exchanges will be vulnerable to data breaches; AI using those sessions to improve algorithms will compromise the long-held ethics around confidentiality in therapy and the associated dangers of personal data being used against clients and therapists. Also, when things go awry, and things always do go awry, it might be difficult to ascertain who is responsible (Atkinson, 2024).

From a pluralistic perspective, a cautious welcome can be offered towards some of the advantages of these technologies. For example, they might offer help to people who, for whatever reasons, may never have been comfortable in a real-life therapeutic relationship. Thus far, however, it is noticeable that, as mentioned earlier, AI is mainly based on CBT and behavioural therapies more generally. This is probably due to CBT's institutional privileges, by being endorsed as 'evidence-based' by bodies such as NICE, but also because the manualised protocols of CBT simplify the process of replicating probable therapist responses to typical client statements and questions. The very nature of relational therapies is based on working with the client to explore problems in ways which may be unpredictable and are expected to be creative and unique. Therapies informed by pluralistic values are, likewise, unpredictable, and therapists who loathe following formulaic protocols and prefer to rely on human interaction are likely to be marginalised by these technologies. Therefore, from a pluralistic perspective, whereby we want to offer people more choice and tailored interventions, AIT is currently coming from a more monist position.

One hope for human therapists is that the personal connection between human beings can never be fully replicated by machines, no matter how advanced or sophisticated (e.g. Cooper, 2024d). This personal connection in therapy is underpinned by an 'I-Thou' attitude in which one subjective being honours the subjectivity of another reciprocally. *Being human* and caring for the other (a machine can only seem like it cares) are essential components of this holistic, relational, intersubjective experience.

Psychedelic Therapy

Another huge 'disruptor' in the therapy field is the gradual normalisation of, and innovations in, the use of psychedelics to enhance personal healing and growth. Psychedelic therapy has a long history (e.g. see Pollan, 2019), but because of an arguably hysterical over-reaction to its potential dangers in the 1960s, there was a long period of near-dormancy from that period until the early 2000s, when a resurgence of psychedelic research in respectable academic and scientific establishments led to what is often called the 'psychedelic renaissance' (e.g. Evans, 2024).

There are still bumps in the road towards integrating psychedelic-assisted therapy as an uncontroversial method. However, I think it is fair to say that the genie is out of the bottle, and with respectable scientists and practitioners proselytising its virtues (as opposed to demonised figures such as Timothy Leary), it will be more challenging to suppress ongoing interest in the therapeutic potentials of psychedelics than it was in the late 1960s and early 1970s.

From a pluralistic perspective, it is important to note that just as there is not one therapy but a multitude of therapies so there is not just one 'psychedelic therapy' but many different angles on how to use psychedelics in therapeutic ways and that variance covers more than just whether they are better used in microdoses, 'heroic' doses, or amounts in between. There is also the danger of psychedelic therapies becoming subsumed by medical systems and medicalisation and the dangers thereof discussed previously. For many at the forefront of the psychedelic renaissance, the movement is not just about mental health interventions or even therapy but deep 'cultural and social transformation' (Evans, 2024). In this respect, those voices echo recent developments in pluralistic therapy, which emphasise the importance of social change as well as personal change and the inextricable synergy of both.

As with any medications, there are risks of harm, and so the professionalised and/or regulated use of psychedelics needs to take these risks into account. Stringent ethical standards need to be applied. Without such safeguards, scandals such as Matthew Perry's ketamine overdose threaten to hinder progress in the development and expansion of psychedelic therapies in treating such conditions as post-traumatic stress disorder (PTSD) (e.g. Birkmayer, 2024). Recently, the BMJ has critiqued the evidence for the benefits of psychedelics as flawed in various ways (BMJ, 2024), and this might be seen as an illustration of the kind of backlash which proponents of psychedelic therapy might expect as they attempt to provide scientific evidence for the benefit of experiences which can only ever be fundamentally subjective and nebulous. I would argue that this is another example of the art/science divide in therapy and the mental health industry more generally.

Pluralism, Therapy, and Mental Health Services

In the UK, therapists watch helplessly as a succession of governments decry the lack of trained and qualified staff for mental health services. At the same time, most are either unemployed (or unpaid in the voluntary sector), underemployed, or resort to the private sector (even when practising in the public sector aligns more congruently with their ideals). According to the BACP, 70% of their members want to work in the NHS and, even with their present non-NHS workloads, could take on the equivalent of one day a week working for the NHS (BACP, 2024a). From a pluralistic perspective, the monistic drive to privilege psychiatrists, psychologists, and a very narrow definition and range of 'psychological' therapists/therapies within the NHS is a hegemonic bulwark that desperately needs to be overcome. The BACP and other professional bodies representing therapists do what they can to ameliorate the situation, but the established powers within the NHS keep on overlooking and devaluing therapists who are willing and able to help people if the gates of the NHS might be opened. With a new Labour government, the readily available, trained and qualified therapist workforce may finally be seen as the obvious solution for more staffing levels rather than reinventing the wheel with a panoply of new titles and trainings.

To a certain extent, the public sector has used the voluntary sector to buoy up the former's lack of provision. There are problems with this development, always there but more so in recent years and especially since the introduction of IAPT (now called Talking Therapies). Issues include the use of trainees and unpaid, qualified therapists to deliver services to some of the most complex and vulnerable people, yet insisting that these same therapists cannot be hired within the NHS because they do not adhere to NHS-approved therapies – a nonsensical double standard. In any case, as economic conditions worsen, many charities find themselves either struggling to survive or having to close (BACP, 2024b). The result is that many people cannot access the help they need either via the NHS or the voluntary sector, with both sectors often having waiting times of months, which, in many cases, is far too long from the point when someone feels the need to either self-refer or be referred. Unless people can afford private fees – expensive but still, on the whole, only allowing therapists modest incomes – they have no access to therapy. This is a situation which leads to unnecessary suffering and, potentially and literally, death and therefore desperately needs to change.

Concluding Thoughts

I am a UK-based therapist. My experience of the therapy field is based on my learning and experiences within a UK context. Agendas around therapy in the UK can only be similar to, and not the same as for therapy internationally. Although the implications of pluralistic philosophies and political theories for therapy might be shared generally across the world, how they manifest in each nation will vary according to specific contexts. For instance, issues around medicalisation and the medical model are shared by practitioners both in the USA and the UK. However, there are significant differences between how the two countries regulate and even conceptualise therapy. For instance, in the USA, therapists are often expected to diagnose their clients, while in the UK, therapists cannot diagnose clients. These medicalised assumptions being embedded in the therapeutic culture cannot help but encourage a more medicalised view of people's problems. So, although the issues raised in this book via looking at therapy through pluralistic lenses have some common ground, how they manifest varies widely from country to country and continent to continent.

Related to diagnoses and medicalisation is the question of medications for mental distress. In the UK, the therapist stance might be best served by being 'neutral' in response to client questions such as 'Do you think I need antidepressants?' My advice is for the client to research the issue for themselves, as all sides of the argument around psychoactive medications are readily available. More recently, however, there has been a move to encourage therapists to flag up more critical takes on antidepressants and their effects: for instance, to inform clients that 'there is no evidence that antidepressants work by correcting a chemical imbalance, that antidepressants have mind-altering effects, and that evidence suggests they produce no noticeable benefit compared with placebo' (Moncrieff, 2018). Currently, in the USA, therapists might be more inclined to encourage the value of medications and psychiatrists. These differences between how therapy manifests in different countries and cultures would be a different book, although distinctly reflective of therapeutic pluralism in terms of psychogeography.

These cultural differences aside, more generally, the pluralistic agenda has implications about which therapies/therapists are offered to whom and how much choice or collaboration clients are allowed. If choice and collaboration are valued – which they might not be (for various reasons) – then the pluralistic agenda is centrally important to how therapy is provided in the future.

Since therapists have significant power in how therapy is 'constructed', how they decide to construct it (which is accomplished at both macrosocial and microsocial levels) is paramount to what is likely to be offered to providers and the public. Of course, therapists have limited power – organisations and 'consumers' themselves interact with what therapists offer and accept or reject those offers. The interactions between these groups can be conceptualised as an ongoing dialogue with empowered and marginalised voices within it. Therapist and client voices are, in particular, somewhat marginalised in cultures that devalue personal, subjective testimony in favour of impersonal, objective evidence.

The most pressing issue related to pluralism and therapy is the increasing marginalisation of a variety (or *plurality*) of different approaches within the NHS and other therapy providers (e.g. BPC/UKCP, 2015). Although pluralistic therapy offers some hope that a greater variety of therapies might be offered to clients/patients in the future, and some campaigning organisations (e.g. Mind and the BACP) openly call for more choice for clients, it is not an unproblematic panacea for the difficulties that many therapies and therapists (and, by implication, clients) currently face.

Dryden (2013), in a chapter in *The Future of Humanistic Psychology* (House et al., 2013), suggests that 'one of the most exciting trends to emerge recently in the field of counselling and psychotherapy has been that of pluralism' (p. 122), and that 'Humanistic Psychology ... should align itself with the pluralistic movement' (pp. 122–123). My ideal for the therapy profession is a future in which professional, economic, and ideological interests cede to a more 'dialogical' approach in which different voices/positions talk with one another, not to dominate or marginalise but rather to understand and negotiate more complex and nuanced positions (e.g. Hermans & Gieser, 2012). For me, this ideal is not just an intellectual, theoretical view but heartfelt and embodied.

There has not been enough consultation with practitioners on a whole range of issues about how to research, professionalise, and regulate the profession. As in other fields, the therapy profession has become victim to top-down thinking and hierarchical directives from institutions that misjudge or dismiss what therapists perceive as the most important elements of practice. One dimension of therapy is to facilitate a sense of empowerment for clients. This is perhaps one reason why such directives face more resistance from psychotherapeutic professionals than other groups.

When I first came across Cooper and McLeod's (2011) book, I perceived it as articulating a version of therapy very close to my perception of my practice. I read the book in a very positive and uncritical way. As the debates about purism versus pluralism raged, I resonated with the pluralistic voices over the purist voices. This was a crucial issue and battle that needed to be fought in the various therapy wars.

I have come, however, to different positions and views. In the first instance, although I am still quite sympathetic to the overall positioning of pluralistic therapy as articulated by Cooper and McLeod, some issues leave me feeling less comfortable.

These issues include discomfort with the apparent 'ownership' of 'pluralistic therapy' by Cooper and McLeod. This ownership was perhaps inevitable as they have produced the most theory and research on the possibilities of 'pluralistic therapy'. However, pluralistic therapy is not something that, by its nature, can be owned or have protocols. To be pluralistic, pluralistic therapists will have a tendency to be suspicious of preordained systems. A pluralistic attitude, in my view, might be summarised in the Blake quotation (spoken by Los in *Jerusalem*), which states 'I must Create a System or be enslav'd by another Man's' (Blake, 1957/1804–1820, p. 629, capitalisation in original). Cooper and McLeod's particular version of 'pluralistic therapy' as a practice is a work-in-progress. It may evolve effectively into frameworks for practice that faithfully reflect the philosophical and political meanings of pluralism, but that point has not yet been reached. Perhaps, following James, that is the nature of attempting to enact the implications of pluralism onto the world of therapy: the attempt will always be 'ever not quite'.

Pluralism, in its philosophical and political meanings, could be most useful in analysing, understanding, and creating the best ways forward for the plurality of therapies and therapists, and the plurality of people and the problems they bring into therapeutic spaces. I trust that I have instigated some understandings of how this might be thought about and progressed into the future.

References

Abertay University (2018). 1st International Conference on Pluralistic Counselling and Psychotherapy: 17–18 March 2018: Book of Abstracts. Accessed at https://www.abertay. ac.uk/media/4233/pluralistic-conf-book-of-abstracts.pdf on 17 March 2018.

ACP (2024). Statement on Statutory Regulation from the Alliance for Counselling & Psychotherapy: November 2024. Accessed at https://allianceblogs.wordpress.com/2024/11/02/ statement-on-statutory-regulation-november-2024/on 18 November 2024.

Addis, M.E., & Jacobson, N.S. (2000). A closer look at the treatment rationale and homework compliance in cognitive-behavioral therapy for depression. *Cognitive Therapy and Research, 24*, 313–326.

Alderdice, J. (2009). *Interview. In S. Aldridge, Counselling – An insecure profession? A sociological and historical analysis* [Doctoral dissertation, University of Leicester].

Aldridge, S. (2011). Counselling – An insecure profession? A sociological and historical analysis [Doctoral dissertation, University of Leicester]. Accessed at https://figshare.le. ac.uk/articles/thesis/Counselling_An_Insecure_Profession_A_Sociological_and_Historical_ Analysis/10103951?file=18213194 on 20 January 2025.

Antoniou, P., Cooper, M., Tempier, A., & Holliday, C. (2017). Helpful aspects of pluralistic therapy for depression. *Counselling and Psychotherapy Research, 17*(2), 137–147.

Araujo, S., & Osbeck, L. (2023). *Ever Not Quite: Pluralism(s) in William James and Contemporary Psychology*. Cambridge: Cambridge University Press.

Arkowitz, H. (1992). Integrative theories of therapy. In D.K. Freedheim (Ed.), *History of Psychotherapy: A Century of Change*. Washington: American Psychological Association.

Atkinson, P. (2024). Machina Ex Deo: AI and the future of NHS Talking Therapies. *The Free Psychotherapy Network*. Accessed at https://freepsychotherapynetwork.com/machina-ex-deo-ai-and-the-future-of-nhs-talking-therapies/ on 22 November 2024.

Ayer, A.J. (1984). *Philosophy in the Twentieth Century*. London: Unwin Paperbacks.

BACP (2009). BACP response to HPC Consultation on the statutory regulation of psychotherapists and counsellors. 9 November 2009. Accessed at http://www.bacp.co.uk/news/? newsld=1603&start=84 on 21 March 2017.

BACP (2010). BACP: Student pages: FAQs: What is the difference between counselling and psychotherapy? Accessed at https://www.bacp.co.uk/student/faq.php on 22 November 2016.

BACP (2017). Results of the 2017 BACP membership survey. Accessed at https://www. bacp.co.uk/about-us/about-bacp/2017-bacp-membership-survey/ on 24 April 2018.

BACP (2024a). Our response to Government's 'Get Britain Working' plans. Accessed at https://www.bacp.co.uk/news/news-from-bacp/2024/27-november-get-britain-working-our-response-to-government-plans/ on 27 November 2024.

BACP (2024b). Vital third sector counselling services need reset of funding relationships. Accessed at https://www.bacp.co.uk/news/news-from-bacp/2024/27-november-vital-third-sector-counselling-services-need-reset-of-funding-relationships/ on 29 November 2024.

Balfour, F. (1995). The British Confederation of Psychotherapists: The background to its establishment and character. Accessed at https://www.bpc.org.uk/resources/history-british-confederation-psychotherapists on 18 November 2016.

Barkham, M., Moller, N.P., & Pybis, J. (2017). How should we evaluate research on counselling and the treatment of depression? A case study on how the National Institute for Health and Care Excellence's draft 2018 guideline for depression considered what counts as best evidence. *Counselling & Psychotherapy Research, 17*(4), 253–268.

Beck, A.T., Rush, A.J., Shaw, B.F., & Emery, G. (1979). *Cognitive Therapy of Depression.* New York: Guilford.

Bell, L.A. (2016). Theoretical foundations for social justice education. In M. Adams, L.A. Bell, D.J. Goodman, & K.Y. Joshi (Eds.), *Teaching for Diversity and Social Justice* (3rd edn., pp. 3–26). London: Routledge.

Bento, W. (2016). Managed mental healthcare in the USA and the care of the soul. In J. Lees (Ed.), *The Future of Psychological Therapy: From Managed Care to Transformational Practice.* Abingdon: Routledge.

Bion, W. (1970). *Attention and Interpretation.* London: Tavistock.

Birkmayer, F. (2024, 11 September). Is the medicine tired? *Befriending the Shadow.* Accessed at https://florianbirkmayermd.substack.com/p/is-the-medicine-tired on 17 November 2024.

Blake, W. (1957/1790–1793). The Marriage of Heaven and Hell. In G. Keynes, *Blake: Complete Writings with Variant Readings.* Oxford: Oxford University Press.

Blake, W. (1957/1804–1820). Jerusalem. In G. Keynes, *Blake: Complete Writings with Variant Readings.* Oxford: Oxford University Press.

Blumer, H. (1986/1969). *Symbolic Interactionism: Perspective and Method.* Berkeley and Los Angeles: University of California Press.

Blunden, N. (2024). Pluralistic person-centred therapy. In M. Cooper (Ed.), *The Tribes of the Person-Centred Nation* (3rd edn., pp. 201–226). Monmouth: PCCS Books.

Blunden, N., Kupfer, C., Smith, K., et al. (2024). Building a community of inquiry for pluralistic practice. *Pluralistic Practice Journal.* https://rke.abertay.ac.uk/en/publications/building-a-community-of-inquiry-for-pluralistic-practice.

BMJ (2024). Analysis: Fragile promise of psychedelics in psychiatry. doi: https://doi.org/10.1136/bmj-2024-080391 (published 19 November 2024).

Boe, T.D., Bertelsen, B., Sundet, R., Hillesund, O.K., & Lidbom, P.A. (2024). Return to reality: What does the world ask of us? *Theory & Psychology, 34*(1), 1–20.

Bohart, A.C. (2000). The client is the most important common factor: Client's self-healing capacities and psychotherapy. *Journal of Psychotherapy Integration, 10*(2), 127–149.

Bohart, A.C., & Tallman, K. (1999). *How Clients Make Therapy Work: The Process of Active Self-Healing.* Washington, D.C.: American Psychological Association.

Bothwell, L.E., & Podolsky, S.H. (2016). The emergence of the randomized, controlled trial. *New England Journal of Medicine, 375,* 501–504. Accessed at http://www.nejm.org/doi/full/10.1056/NEJMp1604635#t=article on 8 November 2016.

Bott, D., & Howard, P. (2012). *The Therapeutic Encounter: A Cross-Modality Approach.* London: Sage.

Boyles, J., & Fathi, N.M. (2019). At what cost? The impact of IAPT on third-sector psychological therapy provision. In C. Jackson & R. Rizq (Eds.), *The Industrialisation of Care: Counselling, Psychotherapy and the Impact of IAPT* (pp. 232–252). Monmouth: PCCS Books.

BPC/UKCP (2015). Addressing the deterioration in public therapy provision. Accessed at https://www.bpc.org.uk/download/1025/PublicPsychotherapyProvision-FINAL.pdf on 10 February 2025.

BPS (2009). History of the British Psychological Society Timeline 1901 to 2009. Accessed at https://cms.bps.org.uk/sites/default/files/2022-06/Timeline%20of%20the%20BPS%201901%20to%202009.pdf on 12 May 2025.

Bradshaw, J. (2024/1990). *Homecoming: Reclaiming and Healing Your Inner Child*. New York: Bantam Books.

Brown, F., & Smith, K. (2023). *Pluralistic Therapy: Responses to Frequently Asked Questions*. London: Routledge.

Bryceland, C., & Stam, H.J. (2018). CBT and empirically validated therapies: Infiltrating codes of ethics. In D. Loewenthal & G. Proctor (Eds.), *Why Not CBT?: Against and For CBT Revisited*. Monmouth: PCCS Books.

Burkeman, O. (2016, 7 January). Therapy wars: The revenge of Freud. *The Guardian*. Accessed at www.theguardian.com/science/2016/jan/07/therapy-wars-revenge-of-freud-cognitive-behavioural-therapy on 18 February 2016.

Butler, S.F., & Strupp, H.H. (1986). Specific and nonspecific factors in psychotherapy: A problematic paradigm for psychotherapy research. *Psychotherapy: Theory, Research, Practice, Training, 23*(1), 30–40. https://doi.org/10.1037/h0085590.

Campbell, D., & Schoolman, M. (Eds.). (2008). *The New Pluralism: William Connolly and the Contemporary Global Condition*. London: Duke University Press.

Cantwell, S. (2018). *Talk about what might be helpful: Relating meta-therapeutic dialogue to concrete interactions and exploring the relevance for therapeutic practice* [Doctoral dissertation, University of Roehampton]. Accessed at https://pure.roehampton.ac.uk/portal/en/studentTheses/talk-about-what-might-be-helpful on 29 August 2024.

Cantwell, S. (2022, 7 April). 'Scaffolding' and 'de-specifying': Deepening an understanding of clients' preferences through conversational analysis. *Pluralistic Practice*. Accessed at https://pluralisticpractice.com/main-blog/training/scaffolding-and-de-specifying-deepening-an-understanding-of-clients-preferences-through-conversational-analysis/ on 27 August 2024.

Carey, T.A. (2005). Can patients specify treatment parameters? A preliminary investigation. *Clinical Psychology and Psychotherapy, 12*, 326–335.

Carey, T.A., & Mullan, R.J. (2007). Patients taking the lead: A naturalistic investigation of a patient-led approach to treatment in primary care. *Counselling Psychology Quarterly, 20*(1), 27–40.

Carrell, S.E. (2001). *The Therapist's Toolbox: 26 Tools and an Assortment of Implements for the Busy Therapist*. London: Sage.

Charura, D., & Winter, L.A. (2023). An introduction to social justice in psychological therapies. In L.A. Winter & D. Charura (Eds.), *The Handbook of Social Justice in Psychological Therapies: Power, Politics, Change*. London: Sage.

Cherniss, J., & Hardy, H. (2023). Isaiah Berlin. In E.N. Zalta & U. Nodelman (Eds.), *The Stanford Encyclopedia of Philosophy (Winter 2023 Edition)*. Accessed at https://plato.stanford.edu/entries/berlin/ as on 20 November 2023.

Clark, J. (Ed.). (2002). *Freelance Counselling and Psychotherapy: Competition and Collaboration*. Hove: Brunner-Routledge.

Clarkson, P. (2003/1995). *The Therapeutic Relationship* (2nd edn.). London: Wiley.

Collins, P.H. (2019). *Intersectionality as Critical Social Theory*. London: Duke University Press.

Collins, P.H., & Bilge, S. (2020). *Intersectionality*. Polity.

Connolly, W.E. (1969). *The Bias of Pluralism*. New York: Atherton.

Connolly, W.E. (2005). *Pluralism*. London: Duke University Press.

Cooper, M. (2007). Humanizing psychotherapy. *Journal of Contemporary Psychotherapy, 37*(1), 11–16.

Cooper, M. (2008). *Essential Research Findings in Counselling and Psychotherapy: The Facts are Friendly*. London: Sage.

Cooper, M. (2015). *Existential Psychotherapy and Counselling: Contributions to a Pluralistic Practice*. London: Sage.

Cooper, M. (2017). Personal correspondence.

Cooper, M. (2019a). *Integrating Counselling and Psychotherapy: Directionality, Synergy & Social Change*. London: Sage.

Cooper, M. (2019b, 9 April). What is pluralism? *Mick Cooper Training and Consultancy*. Accessed at https://mick-cooper.squarespace.com/new-blog/2019/4/9/what-is-pluralism on 18 November 2024.

Cooper, M. (2020, 19 February). Philosophical foundations of pluralism. *Pluralistic Practice*. Accessed at https://pluralisticpractice.com/main-blog/pluralist-philosophy/philosophical-foundations-of-pluralism/ on 12 May 2025.

Cooper, M. (2023). *Psychology at the Heart of Social Change: Developing a Progressive Vision for Society*. Bristol: Policy Press.

Cooper, M. (2024a). *The Tribes of the Person-Centred Nation, Third Edition: An Introduction to the World of Person-Centred Therapies*. Monmouth: PCCS Books.

Cooper, M. (2024b, 10 June). Is person-centred therapy about how we treat people or how we conceptualise people? *Mick Cooper Training and Consultancy*. Accessed at https://mick-cooper.squarespace.com/new-blog/2024/6/10/is-person-centred-therapy-about-how-we-treat-people-or-how-we-conceptualise-people on 22 October 2024.

Cooper, M. (2024c). Progressive social change perspectives and therapy: Mapping the interfaces: Part 1: From progressive social change perspectives to therapy. *Pluralistic Practice*. https://doi.org/10.57064/2164/24580.

Cooper, M. (2024d, 26 November). 'AI-Thou': Can there be relational depth with an AI therapist? *Mick Cooper Training and Consultancy*. Accessed at https://mick-cooper.squarespace.com/new-blog/2024/11/26/ai-thou-can-artificial-intelligence-relate-at-depth on 27 November 2024.

Cooper, M., & Dryden, W. (2016). Introduction. In M. Cooper & W. Dryden (Eds.), *The Handbook of Pluralistic Counselling and Psychotherapy*. London: Sage.

Cooper, M., & McLeod, J. (2007). A pluralistic framework for counselling and psychotherapy: Implications for research. *Counselling and Psychotherapy Research*, 7(3), 135–143.

Cooper, M., & McLeod, J. (2011). *Pluralistic Counselling and Psychotherapy*. London: Sage.

Cooper, M., & McLeod, J. (2012). From either/or to both/and: Developing a pluralistic approach to counselling and psychotherapy. *European Journal of Psychotherapy & Counselling*, 14(1), 5–17.

Cooper, M., Dryden, W., Martin, K., & Papayianni, F. (2016). Metatherapeutic communication and shared decision-making. In M. Cooper & W. Dryden (Eds.), *The Handbook of Pluralistic Counselling and Psychotherapy*. London: Sage.

Cooper, M., McLeod, J., & Smith, K. (2024). Research-informed counselling and psychotherapy: A training and accreditation agenda. *Counselling Psychotherapy Research*, 24(4), 1145–1148. https://doi.org/10.1002/capr.12799.

Cotton, E. (2021, 5 October). The 'Uberisation' of mental health services is a threat to our wellbeing. *The Independent*. Accessed at https://www.independent.co.uk/news/health/mental-health-services-depression-therapy-b1931739.html on 20 May 2024.

Coulter, A., & Collins, A. (2011). *Making Shared Decision-Making a Reality: No Decision About Me, Without Me*. London: The King's Fund.

Curran, J., Parry, G.D., Hardy, G.E., Darling, J., Mason, A-M., & Chambers, E. (2019). How does therapy harm? A model of adverse process using task analysis in the meta-synthesis of service users' experience. *Frontiers in Psychology*, 10, 347. doi: 10.3389/fpsyg.2019.00347.

Cushman, P. (1990). Why the self is empty: Toward a historically situated psychology. *American Psychologist*, 45(5), 599–611.

Cushman, P., & Gilford, P. (1999). From emptiness to multiplicity: The self at the year 2000. *Psychohistory Review*, 27(2), 15–31.

Dalal, F. (2018). *CBT: The Cognitive Behavioural Tsunami: Managerialism, Politics and the Corruptions of Science*. London: Routledge.

Dattilio, F.M., Edwards, D.J.A., & Fishman, D.B. (2010). Case studies within a mixed methods paradigm: Toward a resolution of the alienation between researchers and practitioners in psychotherapy research. *Psychotherapy*, *47*(4), 427–441.

DeAngelis, T. (2010). Closing the gap between practice and research. *Monitor on Psychology*, 41(6). Accessed at https://www.apa.org/monitor/2010/06/gap on 6 September 2024.

de la Prida, A. (2020, 12 May). Bread and jam and sparkling wine? Can I be person-centred and pluralistic? *Pluralistic Practice*. Accessed at https://pluralisticpractice.com/main-blog/personal/bread-and-jam-and-sparkling-wine-can-i-be-person-centred-and-pluralistic/ on 5 February 2025.

Department of Health (2007). *Trust, Assurance and Safety – The Regulation of Health Professionals in the 21st Century*. London: Department of Health.

Department of Health (2008). *Improving Access to Psychological Therapies: Implementation Plan: Curriculum of Low-Intensity Therapies Workers*. London: Department of Health.

Department of Health (2017). *Promoting Professionalism, Reforming Regulation: A Paper for Consultation*. London: Department of Health.

Department of Health and Social Care (2024). Counselling and Psychiatry: Regulation, Question for Department of Health and Social Care, UIN 10097, tabled on 21 October 2024. Accessed at https://questions-statements.parliament.uk/written-questions/detail/2024-10-21/10097 on 18 November 2024.

de Swaan, A. (1990). *The Management of Normality*. London: Routledge.

Drew, C. (2023, 16 August). Cultural pluralism vs multiculturalism (similarities & differences). *Helpful Professor*. Accessed at https://helpfulprofessor.com/cultural-pluralism-vs-multiculturalism/ on 28 November 2023.

Dryden, W. (1999). *Four Approaches to Counselling and Psychotherapy*. Hove: Routledge.

Dryden, W. (2013). Humanistic psychology: Possible ways forward. In R. House, D. Kalisch, & J. Maidman (Eds.), *The Future of Humanistic Psychology*. Ross-on-Wye: PCCS Books.

Duncan, B.L., & Miller, S.D. (2000). The client's theory of change: Consulting the client in the integrative process. *Journal of Psychotherapy Integration*, *10*(2), 169–187. https://doi.org/10.1023/A:1009448200244.

Duncan, E., Best, C., & Hagen, S. (2010). Shared decision making interventions for people with mental health conditions. *Cochrane Database Systematic Review, 1*.

Dunnet, A., Cooper, M., Wheeler, S., Balamoutsou, S., Wilson, C., Hill, A. et al. (2007). Towards Regulation: The Standards, Benchmarks and Training Requirements for Counselling and Psychotherapy. Rugby: BACP.

Ekins, R., & Freeman, R. (Eds.). (1994). *Centres and Peripheries of Psychoanalysis: An Introduction to Psychoanalytic Studies*. London: Karnac Books.

Ellingham, I. (2023). New paradigm person-centred therapy: The reason for practitioners of person-centred therapy to hold onto hope in the face of the 'toxic abominations' of 'person-centred pluralistic therapy', SCoPEd, and psychiatry. Accessed at https://www.ivanellingham.co.uk/images/library/New%20Paradigm%20PCT%201B.pdf on 17 November 2024.

Ellis, A. (1955). New approaches to psychotherapy techniques. *Journal of Clinical Psychology Monograph Supplement*, *11*, 1–53.

Erskine, R.G. (Ed.). (2010). *Life Scripts: A Transactional Analysis of Unconscious Relational Patterns*. London: Karnac Books.

Erskine, R.G., & Moursund, J.P. (2022). *The Art and Science of Relationship: The Practice of Integrative Psychotherapy*. Bicester: Phoenix Publishing House.

Evans, J. (2024, 5 October). Is the psychedelic renaissance over? *Ecstatic Integration*. Accessed at https://www.ecstaticintegration.org/p/is-the-psychedelic-renaissance-over on 8 October 2024.

Eysenck, H.J. (1952). The effects of psychotherapy: An evaluation. *Journal of Consulting Psychology*, *16*(5), 319–324.

Farber, B., & Doolin, E. (2011). Positive regard. *Psychotherapy*, *48*, 58–64.

Feltham, C. (2011/1997). Challenging the core theoretical model. *Counselling*, *8*(2), 121–125; reprinted in R. House & N. Totton (Eds.), *Implausible Professions* (2nd extended edn., pp. 117–128). Ross-on-Wye: PCCS Books.

Feltham, C. (2014). The cultural context of British psychotherapy. In W. Dryden & A. Reeves (Eds.), *The Handbook of Individual Therapy* (6th edn.). London: Sage.

Ferlie, E., Ashburner, L., Fitzgerald, L., & Pettigrew, A. (1996). *New Public Management in Action*. Oxford: Oxford University Press.

Fluckiger, C., Del Re, A.C., Wampold, B.E., & Horvath, A.O. (2018). The alliance in adult psychotherapy: A meta-analytic synthesis. *Psychotherapy*. Advance online publication.

Ford, T. (2024, 8 August). Can therapy survive the AI revolution? *GQ*. Accessed at https://www.gq-magazine.co.uk/article/ai-therapy on 29 November 2024.

Frank, J.D. (1961). *Persuasion and Healing: A Comparative Study of Psychotherapy*. Baltimore: Johns Hopkins University Press.

Frank, J.D., & Frank, J.B. (1991). *Persuasion and Healing: A Comparative Study of Psychotherapy* (3rd edn.). Baltimore: Johns Hopkins University Press.

Frankl, V.E. (1959). *Man's Search for Meaning*. Boston: Beacon Press.

Furedi, F. (2004). *Therapy Culture: Cultivating Uncertainty in an Uncertain Age*. London: Routledge.

Gabriel, L. (2023). Social justice informed therapy and gender. In L.A. Winter & D. Charura (Eds.), *The Handbook of Social Justice in Psychological Therapies: Power, Politics, Change*. London: Sage.

Gergen, K.J. (1990). Therapeutic professions and the diffusion of deficit. *Journal of Mind and Behavior*, *11*(3–4), 353–368.

Gilbert, M., & Orlans, V. (2011). *Integrative Therapy: 100 Key Points and Techniques*. Hove: Routledge.

Gilbert, P., Hughes, W., & Dryden, W. (1989). The therapist as a crucial variable in psychotherapy. In W. Dryden & L. Spurling (Eds.), *On Becoming a Psychotherapist*. London: Routledge.

Goertzen, J.R. (2010). Dialectical pluralism: A theoretical conceptualization of pluralism in psychology. *New Ideas in Psychology*, *28*(2), 201–209.

Goldfried, M.R., Glass, C.R., & Arnkoff, D.B. (2011). Integrative approaches to psychotherapy. In J.C. Norcross, G.E. VanderBos, & D.K. Freedheim, *History of Psychotherapy: Continuity and Change* (2nd edn.). Washington, D.C.: American Psychological Association.

Goodman, D.M. (2016). The McDonaldization of psychotherapy: Processed foods, processed therapies, and economic class. *Theory & Psychology*, *26*(1), 77–95.

Gopaldas, A. (2016). Therapy. *Consumption Markets & Culture*, *19*(3), 264–268.

Grant, A. (2015). Personal communication.

Grogan, J. (2013). *Encountering America: Humanistic Psychology, Sixties Culture & The Shaping of the Modern Self*. New York: HarperCollins.

Hall, R. (2024a, 9 November). 'A therapist shouldn't be giving you hugs': Readers share bad counselling experiences. *The Guardian*.

Hall, R. (2024b, 9 November). MPs urge government to regulate UK psychotherapists and counsellors. *The Guardian*.

Halmos, P. (1965). *The Faith of the Counsellors*. London: Constable.

Hanley, T., & Winter, L.A. (2016). Research and pluralistic counselling and psychotherapy. In M. Cooper & W. Dryden (Eds.), *The Handbook of Pluralistic Counselling and Psychotherapy*. London: Sage.

Hatcher, R.I., & Barends, A.W. (2006). How a return to theory could help alliance research. *Psychotherapy: Theory, Research, Practice, Training*, *43*(3), 293–299.

Hauke, C. (2003/1995). Foreword. In P. Clarkson, *The Therapeutic Relationship* (2nd edn.). London: Wiley.

HCPC (2017). Psychotherapists and counsellors. Accessed at http://www.hcpc-uk.org/aboutregistration/aspirantgroups/psychotherapistscounsellors/ on 15 March 2017.

Hemsley, C. (2013). An enquiry into how counselling psychology in the UK is constructed as a profession within discipline-orientated publications. *Counselling Psychology Review, 28*(1), 8–23.

Hermans, H.J.M., & Gieser, T. (Eds.). (2012). *Handbook of Dialogical Self Theory*. New York: Cambridge University Press.

Hollanders, H. (2014). Integrative therapy. In W. Dryden & A. Reeves (Eds.), *The Handbook of Individual Therapy* (6th edn.). London: Sage.

Hollanders, H., & McLeod, J. (1999). Theoretical orientation and reported practice: A survey of eclecticism among counsellors in Britain. *British Journal of Guidance and Counselling, 27*, 405–414.

Horney, K. (1937). *The Neurotic Personality of Our Time*. London: W.W. Norton.

Horney, K. (1991/1950). *Neurosis and Human Growth: The Struggle Toward Self-Realization*. London: W.W. Norton.

Horvath, A.O., & Greenberg, L.S. (Eds.). (1994). *The Working Alliance: Theory, Research and Practice*. New York: Wiley.

House, R. (2003). *Therapy Beyond Modernity: Deconstructing and Transcending Profession-Centred Therapy*. London: Karnac Books.

House, R. (2011). Pluralistic, post-professional, postmodern? A debate whose time has come. *Letter in Therapy Today, 22*(1). Accessed at http://www.therapytoday.net/article/show/2265/pluralistic-post-professional-postmodern-a-debate-whose-time-has-come/ on 16 November 2015.

House, R. (2016). Beyond the measurable: Alternatives to managed care in research and practice. In J. Lees (Ed.), *The Future of Psychological Therapy: From Managed Care to Transformational Practice*. Abingdon: Routledge.

House, R., Kalisch, D., & Maidman, J. (Eds.). (2013). *The Future of Humanistic Psychology*. Ross-on-Wye: PCCS Books.

House, R., & Totton, N. (Eds.). (1997). *Implausible Professions: Arguments for Pluralism and Autonomy in Psychotherapy and Counselling*. Ross-on-Wye: PCCS Books.

House, R., & Totton, N. (Eds.). (2011). *Implausible Professions: Arguments for Pluralism and Autonomy in Psychotherapy and Counselling* (extended 2nd edn.). Ross-on-Wye: PCCS Books.

HPC (2009). The statutory regulation of psychotherapists and counsellors: Report of the Psychotherapists and Counsellors Professional Liaison Group (PLG) incorporating recommendations to the HPC Council. London: HPC.

Hubble, M.A., Duncan, B.L., & Miller, S.D. (1999). *The Heart and Soul of Change: What Works in Therapy*. Washington, D.C.: American Psychological Association.

Ingersoll, E. (2008). Preface. In A. Marquis, *The Integral Intake: A Guide to Comprehensive Idiographic Assessment in Integral Psychotherapy*. Abingdon: Routledge.

Iwakabe, S. (2003). The pluralistic nature of the field of psychotherapy: A response to Al Mahrer. *Psychology: The Journal of the Hellenic Psychological Society, 10*(1), 25–30.

Jackson, C. (2024). Why Rogers is still relevant. *Therapy Today, 35*(5), 18–23.

James, W. (2011/1908). *A Pluralistic Universe*. Marston Gate: Amazon.co.uk.

Jung, C.G. (1963). *Memories, Dreams, Reflections*. Aniela Jaffe (Ed.). New York: Pantheon.

Kazdin, A.E. (1986). Comparative outcome studies of psychotherapy: Methodological issues and strategies. *Journal of Consulting and Clinical Psychology, 54*, 95–105.

Kelly, P., & Moloney, P. (2018). CBT is the method: The object is to change the heart and soul. In D. Loewenthal & G. Proctor (Eds.), *Why not CBT?: Against and For CBT Revisited*. Monmouth: PCCS Books.

Kiesler, D. (1988). *Therapeutic Metacommunication: Therapist Impact Disclosure as Feedback in Psychotherapy*. Palo Alto: Consulting Psychologists Press.

King, L., & Moutsou, C. (2010). *Rethinking Audit Cultures: A Critical Look at Evidence-Based Practice in Psychotherapy and Beyond*. Ross-on-Wye: PCCS Books.

Kramer, U. (2024). Unifying psychotherapy: Are we there, yet? *Journal of Psychotherapy Integration, 34*(3), 351–355. https://doi.org/10.1037/int0000353.

Lago, C. (2023). Identity and Intersectionality. In L.A. Winter & D. Charura (Eds.), *The Handbook of Social Justice in Psychological Therapies: Power, Politics, Change*. London: Sage.

Laing, R.D. (1960). *The Divided Self: An Existential Study in Sanity and Madness*. Harmondsworth: Penguin.

Lambert, M.J. (1992). Psychotherapy outcome research: Implications for integrative and eclectic practice. In J.C. Norcross & M.R. Goldfried (Eds.), *Handbook of Psychotherapy Integration*. New York: Basic Books.

Larson, M.S. (1977). *The Rise of Professionalism: A Sociological Analysis*. London: University of California Press.

Lassman, P. (2011). *Pluralism*. Cambridge: Polity Press.

Lawton, D., & Nash, S. (2013). The state of humanistic psychology: Where all monkeys are apes but not all apes are monkeys. In R. House, D. Kalisch, & J. Maidman (Eds.), *The Future of Humanistic Psychology*. Ross-on-Wye: PCCS Books.

Lazarus, A.A. (1967). In support of technical eclecticism. *Psychological Reports, 21*, 415–416.

Lazarus, A.A. (1970). *Multimodal Behavior Therapy*. New York: Springer.

Leader, D. (2008, 9 September). A quick fix for the soul? *The Guardian*. Accessed at https://www.theguardian.com/science/2008/sep/09/psychology.humanbehaviour on 31 January 2025.

Leahy, M.J., Rak, E., & Zanskas, S.A. (2015). Chapter 1: A brief history of counseling and specialty areas of practice. In M. Irmo & M.A. Stebnicki (Eds.), *The Professional Counselor's Desk Reference* (2nd edn.). New York: Springer Publishing Company.

Lees, J. (2016). Introduction. In J. Lees (Ed.), *The Future of Psychological Therapy: From Managed Care to Transformational Practice*. London: Routledge.

Lees, J., & Freshwater, D. (Eds.). (2008). *Practitioner-Based Research: Power, Discourse and Transformation*. London: Karnac.

Leite, C., & Kuiper, N.A. (2008). Client uncertainty and the process of change in psychotherapy: The impact of individual differences in self-concept clarity and intolerance of uncertainty. *Journal of Contemporary Psychotherapy, 38*(2), 55–64.

Levinas, E. (1985). *Ethics and Infinity: Conversations with Phillipe Nemo*. Pittsburgh: Duquesne University Press.

Linder, C. (2024, 15 November). Therapy can harm too. *Mad in America*. Accessed at https://www.madinamerica.com/2024/11/therapy-can-harm-too/ on 17 November 2024.

Loewenthal, D. (2011). *Post-Existentialism and the Psychological Therapies: Towards a Therapy without Foundations*. London: Karnac.

Loewenthal, D. (2012). Editorial: pluralism: developments and challenges. *European Journal of Psychotherapy & Counselling, 14*(1), 1–4.

Loewenthal, D. (2016). Therapy as cultural, politically influenced practice. In J. Lees (Ed.), *The Future of Psychological Therapy: From Managed Care to Transformational Practice*. Abingdon: Routledge.

Loewenthal, D., & Proctor, G. (Eds.). (2018). *Why not CBT?: Against and For CBT Revisited*. Monmouth: PCCS Books.

Luborsky, L., Rosenthal, R., Diguer, L., et al. (2002). The Dodo bird verdict is alive and well – mostly. *Clinical Psychology: Science and Practice, 9*(1), 2–12.

Luborsky, L., Singer, B., & Luborsky, L. (1975). Comparative studies of psychotherapies: Is it true that 'Everyone has won and all must have prizes'? *Archive of General Psychiatry, 32*, 995–1008.

Lundh, L-G. (2014). The search for common factors in psychotherapy: Two theoretical models with different empirical implications. *Psychology and Behavioral Sciences*, *3*(5), 131–150. doi: 10.11648/j.pbs.20140305.11.

Lyddon, W.J., & Bradford, E. (1995). Philosophical commitments and therapy approach preferences among psychotherapy trainees. *Journal of Theoretical and Philosophical Psychology*, *15*, 1–15.

Lyotard, J.-F. (1984/1979). *The Postmodern Condition: A Report on Knowledge* (Trans. G. Benningham & B. Massumi). Manchester: Manchester University Press.

Macdonald, K.M. (1995). *The Sociology of the Professions*. London: Sage.

Marquis, A. (2008). *The Integral Intake: A Guide to Comprehensive Idiographic Assessment in Integral Psychotherapy*. Abingdon: Routledge.

Marquis, A. (2024). Unification in psychotherapy: An introduction to the special issue [Editorial]. *Journal of Psychotherapy Integration*, *34*(3), 213–218. https://doi.org/10.1037/int0000351.

Maslow, A.H. (1943). A theory of human motivation. *Psychological Review*, *50*, 370–396.

Maslow, A.H. (1954). *Motivation and Personality*. New York: Harper and Row.

Maslow, A.H. (1968). *Toward a Psychology of Being* (2nd edn.). New York: D. Van Nostrand.

Masson, J. (1992). The tyranny of psychotherapy. In W. Dryden & C. Feltham, *Psychotherapy and Its Discontents*. Buckingham: Open University Press.

Mate, G. (2019). *Scattered Minds: The Origins and Healing of Attention Deficit Disorder*. London: Vermilion.

McAdams, D.P. (1996). Personality, modernity, and the storied self: A contemporary framework for studying persons. *Psychological Inquiry*, *7*(4), 295–321.

McLennan, G. (1995). *Pluralism*. Buckingham: Open University Press.

McLeod, J. (1999). *Practitioner Research in Counselling*. London: Sage.

McLeod, J. (2010). *Case Study Research in Counselling and Psychotherapy*. London: Sage.

McLeod, J. (2013). *An Introduction to Counselling* (5th edn.). Maidenhead: Open University Press.

McLeod, J. (2018). *Pluralistic Therapy: Distinctive Features*. Abingdon: Routledge.

McLeod, J., Smith, K., & Thurston, M. (2016). Training in pluralistic counselling and psychotherapy. In M. Cooper & W. Dryden (Eds.), *The Handbook of Pluralistic Counselling and Psychotherapy*. London: Sage.

McLeod, J., & Sundet, R. (2016). Integrative and eclectic approaches and pluralism. In M. Cooper & W. Dryden (Eds.), *The Handbook of Pluralistic Counselling and Psychotherapy*. London: Sage.

Mearns, D., Thorne, B., & McLeod, J. (2013). *Person-Centred Counselling in Action*. London: Sage.

Metanoia. (2024). BSc (Hons) Person-Centred Pluralistic Counselling (Advanced Practitioner) accessed at https://www.metanoia.ac.uk/programmes/counselling/bsc-hons-person-centred-pluralistic-counselling-advanced-practitioner/ on 9 September 2024.

Michele, A. (2024). Artificial Intelligence is recording your online therapy sessions. *The Ability Toolbox*. Accessed at https://theabilitytoolbox.com/artificial-intelligence-recording-online-therapy/ on 25 November 2024.

Middleton, H. (2015). The medical model: What is it, where does it come from and how long has it got? In D. Loewenthal (Ed.), *Critical Psychotherapy, Psychoanalysis and Counselling: Implications for Practice*. Basingstoke: Palgrave Macmillan.

Miller, S.D., Duncan, B.L., & Hubble, M.A. (1997). *Escape from Babel: Toward a Unifying Language for Psychotherapy Practice*. London: W.W. Norton.

Miller, S.D., Duncan, B.L., Sorrell, R., & Brown, G.S. (2005). The partners for change outcome management system. *Journal of Clinical Psychology*, *61*(2), 199–208.

Mills, C.W. (1956). *The Power Elite*. Oxford University Press.

Milne, A. (2003). *Teach Yourself Counselling*. London: Hodder Arnold.

Mind (2013). *We Still Need to Talk: A Report on Access to Talking Therapies*. London: Mind.

Molyneux, C. (2014). The problem with pluralism. *Therapy Today, 25*(4), 32–33.

Molyneux, C. (2024, 21 October). What is an approach to counselling and who defines it? The risks of postmodernism and pluralism in person-centred counselling. *Chris the Counsellor*. Accessed at https://christhecounsellor.co.uk/pluralism-and-the-person-centred-approach/ on 22 October 2024.

Moncrieff, J. (2018). Against the stream: Antidepressants are not antidepressants – An alternative approach to drug action and implications for the use of antidepressants. *BJPsych Bulletin, 42*(1), 42–44. doi:10.1192/bjb.2017.11.

Montgomery, A. (2013). *Neurobiology Essentials for Clinicians: What Every Therapist Needs to Know*. New York: Norton.

Morgan-Ayrs, S. (2016). Regulation, institutionalized ethics and the therapeutic frame. In J. Lees (Ed.), *The Future of Psychological Therapy: From Managed Care to Transformational Practice*. Abingdon: Routledge.

Muasher, M. (2014). Pluralism is necessary for democracy. NPR's Diane Rehm Show, 20 February 2014. Accessed at https://carnegieendowment.org/2014/02/20/pluralism-is-necessary-for-democracy-pub-54609 on 17 January 2024.

NCPS (2024). *Therapeutic Relationships: The Human Connection*. https://ncps.com'about-us'campaigns/therapeutic-relationships-the-human-connection.

Norcross, J.C. (Ed.). (2002). *Psychotherapy Relationships that Work: Therapist Contributions and Responsiveness to Patients*. Oxford: Oxford University Press.

Norcross, J.C. (2011). *Psychotherapy Relationships that Work: Evidence-Based Responsiveness*. New York: Oxford University Press.

Norcross, J.C. (2023). Personal communication.

Norcross, J.C., & Cooper, M. (2021). *Personalizing Psychotherapy: Assessing and Accommodating Patient Preferences*. Washington: American Psychological Association.

Norcross, J.C., & Goldfried, M.R. (Eds.). (1992). *Handbook of Psychotherapy Integration*. New York: Basic Books.

Norcross, J.C., & Goldfried, M.R. (2005). *Handbook of Psychotherapy Integration* (2nd edn.). Oxford: Oxford University Press.

Norcross, J.C., Karpiak, C.P., & Lister, K.M. (2005). What's an integrationist? A study of self-identified integrative and (occasionally) eclectic psychologists. *Journal of Clinical Psychology, 61*, 1587–1594.

Norcross, J.C., & Lambert, M.J. (2011a). Psychotherapy relationships that work II. *Psychotherapy, 48*(1), 4–8.

Norcross, J.C., & Lambert, M.J. (2011b). Evidence-based therapy relationships. In J.C. Norcross (Ed.), *Psychotherapy Relationships That Work: Evidence-Based Responsiveness* (2nd edn.). New York: Oxford University Press.

Norcross, J.C., & Lambert, M.J. (2019). *Psychotherapy Relationships That Work: Volume 1: Evidence-Based Therapist Contributions* (3rd edn.). New York: Oxford University Press.

Norcross, J.C., & Saltzman, N. (1990). The clinical exchange: Toward integrating the psychotherapies. In N. Saltzman & J.C. Norcross (Eds), *Therapy Wars: Contention and Convergence in Differing Clinical Approaches*. San Francisco: Jossey-Bass.

Norcross, J.C., VanderBos, G.E., & Freedheim, D.K. (2011). *History of Psychotherapy: Continuity and Change* (2nd edn.). Washington, D.C.: American Psychological Association.

Norcross, J.C., & Wampold, B.E. (2018). A new therapy for each patient: Evidence-based relationships and responsiveness. *Journal of Clinical Psychology, 74*(11), 1889–1906. doi: 10.1002/jclp.22678.

O'Connell, B. (2005). *Solution-Focused Therapy* (2nd edn.). London: Sage.

Ong, W.T., Murphy, D., & Joseph, S. (2020). Unnecessary and incompatible: A critical response to Cooper and McLeod's conceptualization of a pluralistic framework for person-centered therapy. *Person-Centered & Experiential Psychotherapies, 19*(2), 168–182. doi.org/10.1080/14779757.2020.1717987.

Orlans, V., & Van Scoyoc, S. (2009). *A Short Introduction to Counselling Psychology*. London: Sage.

Owen, J., & Hilsenroth, M.J. (2014). Treatment adherence: The importance of therapist flexibility in relation to therapy outcomes. *Journal of Counseling Psychology, 61*, 280–288.

Owens, M. (2014). Against factionalism. *Therapy Today, 25*(4), 28–31.

Papayianni, F., & Cooper, M. (2017). Metatherapeutic communication: An exploratory analysis of therapist-reported moments of dialogue regarding the nature of the therapeutic work. *British Journal of Guidance & Counselling, 46*(2), 173–184. doi: 10.1080/03069885.2017.1305098.

Parker, I. (Ed.). (1999a). *Deconstructing Psychotherapy*. London: Sage.

Parker, I. (1999b). Deconstruction and psychotherapy. In I. Parker (Ed.), *Deconstructing Psychotherapy*. London: Sage.

Parker, I. (2015). *Psychology after Lacan: Connecting the Clinic and Research*. Hove: Routledge.

Perls, F.S., Hefferline, R.F., & Goodman, P. (1951). *Gestalt Therapy: Excitement and Growth in the Human Personality*. New York: Julian Press.

Pilgrim, D., Rogers, A., & Bentall, R. (2009). The centrality of personal relationships in the creation and amelioration of mental health problems: The current interdisciplinary case. *Health: An Interdisciplinary Journal for the Social Study of Health, Illness and Medicine, 13*(2), 235–254.

Pinker, S. (2019). *Enlightenment Now: The Case for Reason, Science, Humanism, and Progress*. London: Penguin.

Plato (2003/1954). *The Last Days of Socrates* (Trans. H. Tredennick & H. Tarrant). London: Penguin.

Polkinghorne, D.E. (1992). Postmodern epistemology of practice. In S. Kvale (Ed.), *Psychology and Postmodernism*. London: Sage.

Pollan, M. (2019). *How to Change Your Mind: The New Science of Psychedelics*. London: Penguin Books.

Poole, J. (2024, 10 October). Letters: We need person-centred mental health care, not more psychiatrists. *The Guardian*. Accessed at https://www.theguardian.com/society/2024/oct/10/we-need-person-centred-mental-health-care-not-more-psychiatrists on 12 October 2024.

Proctor, G. (2016). Book review: Critical Psychotherapy, Psychoanalysis and Counselling: Implications for Practice, Ed. D. Loewenthal. *Counselling and Psychotherapy Research, 16*(2), 145–146.

Purton, C. (2016). Why the Dodo got it right. *Therapy Today, 27*(1), 24–27.

Pybis, J., Saxon, D., Hill, A., & Barkham, M. (2017). The comparative effectiveness and efficiency of cognitive behaviour therapy and generic counselling in the treatment of depression: Evidence from the 2nd UK National Audit of psychological therapies. *BMC Psychiatry, 17*(215). Accessed at https://bmcpsychiatry.biomedcentral.com/articles/10.1186/s12888-017-1370-7 on 9 August 2017.

Rabu, M., & McLeod, J. (2018). Wisdom in professional knowledge: Why it can be valuable to listen to the voices of senior psychotherapists. *Psychotherapy Research, 28*(5), 776–792.

Reeves, A. (2014). Research in individual therapy. In W. Dryden & A. Reeves (Eds.), *The Handbook of Individual Therapy* (6th edn.). London: Sage.

Reid, A.J. (2002, 8 May). Trade unions: A foundation of political pluralism? *History & Policy*. Accessed at https://www.historyandpolicy.org/policy-papers/papers/trade-unions-a-foundation-of-political-pluralism on 17 January 2024.

Rennie, D.L. (1994). Clients' deference in psychotherapy. *Journal of Counselling Psychology, 41*(4), 427–437.

Rennie, D.L. (1998). *Person-Centred Counselling: An Experiential Approach*. London: Sage.

Rescher, N. (1993). *Pluralism: Against the Demand for Consensus*. Oxford: Oxford University.

Rhodes, J., & Smith, J.A. (2010). 'The top of my head came off': An interpretative phenomenological analysis of the experience of depression. *Counselling Psychology Quarterly, 23*(4), 399–409.

Riddle, A. (2024, 26 June). Unmasking the politics behind CBT's rise to prominence. *Mad in America*. Accessed at https://www.madinamerica.com/2024/06/unmaking-the-politics-behind-cbts-rise-to-prominence on 28 June 2024.

Ritzer, G. (2015). *The McDonaldization of Society* (8th edn.). London: Sage.

Rizq, R. (2016). States of abjection in managed care. In J. Lees (Ed.), *The Future of Psychological Therapy: From Managed Care to Transformational Practice*. Abingdon: Routledge.

Robb, A. (2024, 2 March). 'He checks in on me more than my friends and family': Can AI therapists do better than the real thing? *The Guardian*. Accessed at https://www.theguardian.com/lifeandstyle/2024/mar/02/can-ai-chatbot-therapists-do-better-than-the-real-thing on 22 November 2024.

Robson, C. (2011). *Real World Research: A Resource for Users of Social Research Methods in Applied Settings* (3rd edn.). Chichester: John Wiley & Sons.

Rogers, C.R. (1942). *Counseling and Psychotherapy*. New York: Houghton Mifflin.

Rogers, C.R. (2003/1951). *Client-Centered Therapy: Its Current Practice, Implications and Theory*. London: Constable.

Rogers, C.R. (1957). The necessary and sufficient conditions of psychotherapeutic personality change. *Journal of Consulting Psychology, 21*, 95–103.

Rogers, C.R. (1961). *On Becoming a Person: A Therapist's View of Psychotherapy*. London: Constable.

Rogers, C.R. (1980). *A Way of Being*. New York: Houghton Mifflin.

Rorty, R. (1991). *Objectivity, Relativism, and Truth*. Cambridge: Cambridge University Press.

Rosenthal, D., & Frank, J.D. (1956). Psychotherapy and the placebo effect. *Psychological Bulletin, 53*, 294–302.

Rosenzweig, S. (1936). Some implicit common factors in diverse methods of psychotherapy: 'At last the Dodo said, "Everybody has won and all must have prizes"'. *American Journal of Orthopsychiatry, 6*, 412–415.

Rowan, J. (2005a). *The Transpersonal: Spirituality in Psychotherapy and Counselling* (2nd edn.) Hove: Routledge.

Rowan, J. (2005b). *The Future of Training in Psychotherapy and Counselling: Instrumental, Relational and Transpersonal Perspectives*. Hove: Routledge.

Rowan, J. (2015). Personal communication.

Rowan, J. (2016). *The Reality Game: A Guide to Humanistic Counselling and Psychotherapy* (3rd edn.) Abingdon: Routledge.

Rowan, J., & Cooper, M. (1998). *The Plural Self: Multiplicity in Everyday Life*. London: Sage.

Rowan, J., & Glouberman, D. (2018). What is humanistic psychology? In R. House, D. Kalisch, & J. Maidman (Eds.), *Humanistic Psychology: Current Trends and Future Prospects*. Abingdon: Routledge.

Royal College of Psychiatrists. How effective is CBT? Accessed at https://www.rcpsych.ac.uk/mental-health/treatments-and-wellbeing/cognitive-behavioural-therapy-(cbt) on 8 July 2024.

Russell, B. (1959). *My Philosophical Development*. London: George Allen & Unwin.

Sackett, D.L., Rosenberg, W.M., Gray, J.A.M., Haynes, R.B., & Richardson, W.S. (1996). Evidence based medicine: What it is and what it isn't. *British Medical Journal, 312*, 71–72.

Safran, J.D., & Messer, S.B. (1997). Psychotherapy integration: A postmodern critique. *Clinical Psychology: Science and Practice, 4*(2), 140–152.

Saltzman, N., & Norcross, J.C. (Eds). (1990). *Therapy Wars: Contention and Convergence in Differing Clinical Approaches*. San Francisco: Jossey-Bass.

Samuels, A. (2011/1997). Pluralism and psychotherapy: What is a good training? In R. House & N. Totton (Eds.), *Implausible Professions: Arguments for Pluralism and Autonomy in Psychotherapy and Counselling*. Ross-on-Wye: PCCS Books.

Sanders, P. (Ed.). (2012). *The Tribes of the Person-Centred Nation: An Introduction to the Schools of Therapy Related to the Person-Centred Approach*. Ross-on-Wye: PCCS Books.

Schoolman, D., & Campbell, D. (2008a). Introduction: Pluralism 'Old' and 'New'. In D. Campbell & M. Schoolman (Eds.), *The New Pluralism: William Connolly and the Contemporary Global Condition*. London: Duke University Press.

Schoolman, D., & Campbell, D. (2008b). An interview with William Connolly, December 2006. In D. Campbell & M. Schoolman (Eds.), *The New Pluralism: William Connolly and the Contemporary Global Condition*. London: Duke University Press.

Schwarz, R.J.C. (1995). *Internal Family Systems Therapy*. New York: The Guilford Press.

Scott, A.J., & Hanley, T. (2012). On becoming a pluralistic therapist: A case study of a student's reflexive journal. *Counselling Psychology Review, 27*(4), 28–40.

Scott, S. (2015). *Negotiating Identity: Symbolic Interactionist Approaches to Social Identity*. Cambridge: Polity Press.

Shepherd, M., Evans, C., Ashworth, M., Nairne, K., & Robinson, S.I. (2007). Making CORE-OM data work for you and your service: A primary care psychology and counselling team's experience of routine outcome measurement. *Clinical Psychology Forum, 174*, 31–34.

Skills for Health (2017). Person-centred approaches: Empowering people in their lives and communities to enable an upgrade in prevention, wellbeing, health, care and support: A core skills education and training framework. Accessed at https://www.skillsforhealth.org.uk/resources/person-centred-approaches-2017/ on 2 December 2024.

Skinner, B.F. (1953). *Science and Human Behavior*. New York: The Free Press.

Smail, D. (2005). *Power, Interest and Psychology: Elements of a Social Materialist Understanding of Distress*. Ross-on-Wye: PCCS Books.

Smith, K., & de la Prida, A. (2021). *The Pluralistic Therapy Primer: A Concise Introduction*. PCCS Books Ltd: Monmouth.

Sparks, J.A., & Duncan, B.L. (2016). Client strengths and resources: Helping clients draw on what they already do best. In M. Cooper & W. Dryden (Eds.), *The Handbook of Pluralistic Counselling and Psychotherapy*. London: Sage.

Spinelli, E. (1996). Do therapists know what they're doing? In I. James & S. Palmer (Eds.), *Professional Therapeutic Titles: Myths and Realities*. Leicester: British Psychological Society, Div. Couns. Psychol., Occasional Paper 2.

SPR. (2022). Stakeholder position statement on the NICE guideline for depression in adults. Accessed at https://cdn.ymaws.com/www.psychotherapyresearch.org/resource/resmgr/uk-spr/spruk_nice_01_2022.pdf on 21 January 2025.

Spring, B. (2007). Evidence-based practice in clinical psychology: What it is, why it matters; what you need to know. *Journal of Clinical Psychology, 63*(7), 611–632.

Spurling, L. (2016). Psychodynamic approaches and pluralism. In M. Cooper & W. Dryden (Eds.), *The Handbook of Pluralistic Counselling and Psychotherapy*. London: Sage.

Stam, H.J. (2023). Foreword. In S. Araujo & L. Osbeck, *Ever Not Quite: Pluralism(s) in William James and Contemporary Psychology*. Cambridge: Cambridge University Press.

Stiles, W.B., Shapiro, D.A., & Elliott, R. (1986). Are all psychotherapies equivalent? *American Psychologist, 41*, 165–180.

Storm, J.A.J. (2021). *Metamodernism: The Future of Theory*. Chicago: University of Chicago Press.

Sundet, R., & McLeod, J. (2016). Narrative approaches and pluralism. In M. Cooper & W. Dryden (Eds.), *The Handbook of Pluralistic Counselling and Psychotherapy*. London: Sage.

Swift, J.K., Callahan, J.L., & Vollmer, B.M. (2011). Preferences. In J.C. Norcross (Ed.), *Psychotherapy Relationships that Work* (2nd edn.). New York: Oxford University Press.

Szasz, T. (1960). The myth of mental illness. *American Psychologist, 15*, 113–118.

Szasz, T. (1961). *The Myth of Mental Illness: Foundations of a Theory of Personal Conduct.* New York: Hoeber-Harper.

Szasz, T. (1988). *The Myth of Psychotherapy: Mental Healing as Religion, Rhetoric and Repression* (2nd edn.). Syracuse: Syracuse University Press.

Talley, P.F., Strupp, H.H., & Butler, S.F. (1994). *Psychotherapy Research and Practice: Bridging the Gap.* New York: Basic Books.

Tallis, R. (2011). *Aping Mankind: Neuromania, Darwinitis and the Misrepresentation of Humanity.* Durham: Acumen.

Task Force on Promotion and Dissemination of Psychological Procedures (1995). Training in and dissemination of empirically-validated psychological treatment: Report and recommendations. *Clinical Psychologist, 48*, 2–23.

Theriault, A., & Gazzola, N. (2006). What are the sources of feelings of incompetence in experienced therapists? *Counselling Psychology Quarterly, 19*(4), 313–330.

Theriault, A., & Gazzola, N. (2008). Feelings of incompetence among experienced therapists: A substantive theory. *European Journal of Qualitative Research in Psychotherapy, 4*, 19–29.

Thoma, N.C., & Cecero, J.J. (2009). Is integrative use of techniques in psychotherapy the exception or the rule? Results of a national survey of doctoral-level practitioners. *Psychotherapy, 46*(4), 405–417.

Thompson, A., & Cooper, M. (2012). Therapists' experiences of pluralistic practice. *European Journal of Psychotherapy & Counselling, 14*(1), 63–75.

Thornton, J. (2018). Depression in adults: Campaigners and doctors demand full revision of NICE guidance. *British Medical Journal, 361*. Accessed at https://www.bmj.com/content/361/bmj.k2681 on 17 July 2018.

Tudor, K. (2018a). *Psychotherapy: A Critical Examination.* Monmouth: PCCS Books.

Tudor, K. (2018b). From humanism to humanistic psychology and back again. In R. House, D. Kalisch, & J. Maidman (Eds.), *Humanistic Psychology: Current Trends and Future Prospects.* Abingdon: Routledge.

Turner, D. (2021). *Intersections of Privilege and Otherness in Counselling and Psychotherapy: Mockingbird.* London: Routledge.

Turner, D. (2024). *The Psychology of Supremacy: Imperium.* Abingdon: Routledge.

UK Parliament (2019). Counsellors and Psychotherapists (Regulation) and Conversion Therapy Bill 2017–2019. Accessed at https://bills.parliament.uk/bills/2284 on 20 January 2025.

Walker, C., Hanna, P., & Hart, A. (2015). Psychology without psy professionals: Exploring an unemployed centre families project as a mental health resource. *Journal of Community & Applied Social Psychology, 25*(1), 502–512.

Waller, D. (2009). Psychotherapy in Europe: An emerging professional project. *European Journal of Psychotherapy & Counselling, 11*(2), 203–209.

Wampold, B.E. (2010). The research evidence for common factors: A historically situated position. In B.L. Duncan, S.D. Miller, B.E. Wampold, & M.A. Hubble (Eds.), *The Heart and Soul of Change: Delivering What Works in Therapy* (2nd edn.). Washington, D.C.: American Psychological Association.

Wampold, B.E. (2022). Dr. Bruce Wampold on how to make therapy better. Interview accessed at https://www.jordanthecounselor.com/post/bruce-wampold-interview on 21 October 2024.

Wampold, B.E., & Bhati, K.S. (2004). Attending to the omissions: A historical examination of evidence-based practice movements. *Professional Psychology: Research and Practice, 35*(6), 563–570.

Wampold, B.E., & Imel, Z.E. (2015). *The Great Psychotherapy Debate: The Evidence for What Makes Therapy Work* (2nd edn.). Hove: Routledge.

Ward, J. (1911). *The Realm of Ends, or Pluralism and Theism*. Cambridge: Cambridge University Press.

Watson, G. (1940). Areas of agreement in psychotherapy. *American Journal of Orthopsychiatry, 10*, 698–709.

Watson, V.C., Cooper, M., McArthur, K., & McLeod, J. (2012). Helpful therapeutic processes: Client activities, therapist activities and helpful effects. *European Journal of Psychotherapy & Counselling, 14*(1), 77–89.

Wenger, E. (1997). *Communities of Practice: Learning, Meaning and Identity*. New York: Cambridge University Press.

White, M., & Epston, D. (1990). *Narrative Means to Therapeutic Ends*. London: W.W. Norton.

Wilber, K. (1979). *No Boundary*. Los Angeles: Center Publications.

Wilber, K. (2000). *Integral Psychology: Consciousness, Spirit, Psychology, Therapy*. Boston: Shambhala Publications.

Wilson, L. (2024). Reactions. *Therapy Today, 35*(6), 13.

Wolpe, J. (1958). *Psychotherapy by Reciprocal Inhibition*. Stanford: Stanford University Press.

Woods, D. (2009). *Beginning Postmodernism*. Manchester: Manchester University Press.

Yalom, I.D. (2015). *Creatures of a Day: And Other Tales of Psychotherapy*. New York: Basic Books.

Index

For Product Safety Concerns and Information please contact our EU
representative GPSR@taylorandfrancis.com
Taylor & Francis Verlag GmbH, Kaufingerstraße 24, 80331 München, Germany